D0401704

SEE
MOM
RUN

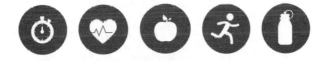

EVERY MOTHER'S GUIDE
TO GETTING FIT AND

RUNNING HER FIRST 5K

Megan Searfoss

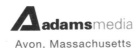
Aadamsmedia

Avon, Massachusetts

Published by
Adams Media, a division of F+W Media, Inc.
57 Littlefield Street, Avon, MA 02322. U.S.A.
www.adamsmedia.com

ISBN 10: 1-4405-7577-0
ISBN 13: 978-1-4405-7577-8
eISBN 10: 1-4405-7578-9
eISBN 13: 978-1-4405-7578-5

Printed in the United States of America.

10   9   8   7   6   5   4   3   2   1

Many of the designations used by manufacturers and sellers to distinguish their products are
claimed as trademarks. Where those designations appear in this book and F+W Media, Inc.
was aware of a trademark claim, the designations have been printed with initial capital letters.

The information in this book should not be used for diagnosing or treating any health problem.
Not all diet and exercise plans suit everyone. You should always consult a trained medical
professional before starting a diet, taking any form of medication, or embarking on any fitness
or weight-training program. The author and publisher disclaim any liability arising directly or
indirectly from the use of this book.

Cover design by Stephanie Hannus.
Cover images © soleilc1/123RF; Justin Roque/123RF.

This book is available at quantity discounts for bulk purchases.
For information, please call 1-800-289-0963.

Dedication

This book is dedicated to Noreen,
Queen Mother of the Hill,
Always a mother, always a runner, always my friend.
"I believe I can fly."

Acknowledgments

Thousands of women have contributed to *See Mom Run*, and knowingly and unknowingly they have influenced my words and will inspire you to take the steps toward your running life.

Thank you to the Ridgefield Racy Ladies—my beloved running group who have shared their thoughts, stories, and miles with me for years and continue to be the reason I wake up at the crack of dawn on Sunday. They are the motivation behind the start of Run Like a Mother, a little hometown race that celebrates who we are as women, mothers, and runners. Our lives are forever connected through incredible ups and downs, and it is our running that has strengthened our hearts and souls.

Thank you to the hundreds of women who shared their love of running with me. Their candid comments about why they started to run, their struggles, and their triumphs will encourage you to lace up and step out. Their stories are encouraging and real.

I am grateful to the thousands of women who toe the line every year at Run Like a Mother races across the country. Their commitment to running not only improves their lives but also shows the importance of "me time" and teaches their children how to live healthy, train for a goal, and reach it. These women have learned to run through my training programs and have shared with me valuable insights—through which I have learned what works for moms in every stage of life.

And most importantly, my family who challenge me to Run Like a Mother every day. Their support of my passion continues to push me as much as I encourage them to live life fully despite their own challenges. Chon, Abby, Sarah, and Jane, your strength is my inspiration. I love you. Run on!

Introduction

Endless studies extol the virtues of running. It improves your cardio-vascular fitness, sculpts legs, hones your core, and invigorates your mind. Done on a regular basis, it can even help you fit into those "skinny" jeans you have tucked into the back of your closet for the day when you're back to your fighting weight. Running is inexpensive (no fancy equipment required!), and something you can do almost anywhere, so it is perfect for a mom who usually is running for everyone but herself. Yet many of us remain intimidated by the idea of joining the growing ranks of runners throughout the country. We don't see ourselves as athletes, or runners. But why not? What's stopping us? And, most importantly, where do we start?

Running is an incredible resource for fitness and "me time." It may not always seem like you have the time, but I promise you that every mother has it in her to run for fitness, for fun, or for friendship. This book will arm you with the technical advice you need to get started, inspire you with some "you go girl" enthusiasm, and give you the confidence you deserve to become a runner. You can run, you will run, and you may even convert your closest friends.

Let's be honest; there are always reasons not to start running: You've just had a baby, you drive five carpools, you are delicately balancing work and family, and the laundry is on an endless cycle of wash, re-wash and unwrinkle. If you've picked up this book, it means you are searching for reasons to get started, and there are many. Maybe you're looking for a convenient way to get fit, or lose lingering baby weight. Maybe you have seen women running together and are looking for a more social exercise. Or perhaps you are intrigued by the challenge of a 5K race after hearing others talk about how much fun they have had with the distance. No matter what your reasons, you'll find this book to be an easy resource for getting yourself motivated, training, and running. There are individual training programs, meant for women at different ability levels. You pick the one that works best for you, your schedule, and your family:

- **Creeping:** Making the Time and Preparing the Body to Run by Walking
- **Crawling:** Building the Run with Run/Walk Intervals
- **Cruising:** Running Throughout the Workout
- **Climbing:** Running Competitively

I remember clearly the day I made the decision to become a runner. I stepped out the door to take those first baby steps, and no one was there to cheer, video, or photograph me (and for that I am thankful). I was a new mom with a job outside the home. I was bleary-eyed and sleep deprived with no time to exercise, but I realized I desperately needed to make time for myself. It wasn't easy, and, in fact, there were many times starting out when I felt defeated and embarrassed. Running felt too hard, too awkward, and too exhausting.

I kept running, and then gradually it happened—I started to notice that running relieved my stress and made me feel healthier; I slept better and my outlook on our new crazy family life was brighter. I made time to run and my life magically gained time. I suddenly had the energy to do all the things that needed to get done. My body began to adapt and respond too. I was leaner, stronger, and soon I craved the exhilarating feeling that running gave me.

See Mom Run is meant to help you find that feeling too. Running can be difficult when you're starting out, so together we will deconstruct and demystify the exercise to make it more understandable and, best yet, achievable. This book is meant to give you the inspiration to keep running when you just don't feel like it, the motivation even when it's hard, and perspiration it takes for you to be the best you can be. You will discover the benefits of running, and learn what kind of gear you need, and how simple reminders of form will help you move your body the way it was meant to run. We'll talk about the motivation to find the time away from the kids (or even with the kids) and to get out the door. Even if you have never run or exercised before, my tried-and-true 5K training guides will help you feel ready and able to finish a 5K. And then we will cross the finish line together, and help you find your groove as both a mother and a runner.

Running can be an individual or a social exercise. It can be fast or conversational. It benefits your legs and lungs, but also your mind and spirit. It will carry you through some of the lowest points in your life and then lift you up to your greatest personal accomplishments. Running is sometimes drudgery, but mostly pure joy. You will never regret a run though you might regret not running.

Running has made me a better person, wife, mother, friend, but most importantly, a better self, and it will do the same for you. Surprisingly, as a mom, when I thought there was not an extra minute in the day, running created time. I hope by reading *See Mom Run* you will find the joy of running and reconnect with the feeling you experienced as a child. Whether it is for fitness, fun, friendship, or to run your first 5K, it shouldn't be daunting or scary to run because, after all, it's who we are and it's what we do. Run Like a Mother, like you already do, but this time make it for you.

PART 1

See Mom Run

"Running is the greatest metaphor for life,
because you get out of it what you put into it."

—Oprah Winfrey

CHAPTER 1

The Benefits of Running

Magical things happen when you become a runner. Some changes you will see: Your clothes will fit better and your body will feel firmer. But it also affects you in more subtle ways. You just feel different— happier, more confident, and energetic. Running challenges your mind and body in ways you can't imagine at first, and then it becomes a predictable, steady friend you can count on. Its benefits and effects are varied and endless, as every outing can provide a different challenge as terrain, miles, distance, and years go by.

During our overscheduled lives, as moms we may feel that taking even a sliver of time for ourselves is selfish and irresponsible. If that sliver comes, certainly there is something you must have missed: a school project deadline, a PTA meeting, or the laundry that never seems to be done. You are pulled in twenty different "mom" directions every day, leaving no time for you. How could you possibly fit running into your schedule?

The truth is that everyone feels this way when they're getting started. It's worth it to carve out that time, because the benefits of running are truly greater than simply strengthening the legs that propel you. Your mind, your time, and your family will benefit. It may sound incredulous to say that simply moving your feet will change your world, but it will. The running time you take, even if it's only a small part of your week, will positively influence the rest of your day and change your life in wonderful, healthy ways.

Through this book, I won't intimidate you with discussions of mitochondria, adenosine triphosphate, lactate threshold, or macrocycles, and I won't insist you buy anything more than a supportive bra, non-cotton socks, real running shoes, a chronograph watch for running, and a stability ball for strength training. I can't guarantee you dramatic weight loss or a Boston Marathon–qualifying run, because that's not what this book is intended to do. I can promise you, though, that if you give running a chance, you will prime your body to be capable of doing whatever you set out to do. Running doesn't discriminate. There is no single body type, no specific pace, or stay-at-home versus working-mom requisite. Running is an individual exercise that knows no time boundary, no membership fee, and no crazy routine to follow in front of unforgiving mirrors and blaring music. It will help you become healthier and leaner, and more confident. You will stand taller, and best of all, you will think more clearly.

THE PHYSICAL BENEFITS OF RUNNING

Most people begin running for the physical benefits: to improve muscle tone, for overall health, and mostly for what I like to call "jeans therapy." Blame weight gain on your babies, getting older, hormones, or a lazy metabolism, but the truth is that as we become adults we move our bodies less and lose precious muscle tone. If fitting into those pre-baby jeans is your primary motivation to start (whether that baby is six months or twenty-two years old), that's definitely not a bad thing.

Have you ever tried to move like your two-year-old? Or even your seven-year-old? The chances are that you aren't moving as much as you did ten years ago. Don't curse a sluggish or aging metabolism. Fight back and change the numbers. Running is a great choice for an exercise, as it offers the highest calorie burn per minute compared to any other physical activity, other than cross-country skiing. Opting to use diet only as a weight-loss tool will leave you with little energy to care for the kids and will drive you crazy. Running will help you lose post-baby pounds and then stabilize your weight, as the increased muscle tone and mass will enable your body to burn more calories. Weight loss is wonderful, but it's far from the only reason you should lace up and head out. The overall health benefits of running are compelling and reason enough to fit it in.

Enhance Your Chest

Running won't make your breasts larger, but it definitely benefits those two balloon-type organs inside your chest: your lungs. The American Lung Association says: "the lung is healthier the more it is exercised. For people with asthma, strengthening their lungs will mean that they will be better able to deal with their asthma, physically." As you incorporate running into your life, your respiratory system becomes much more efficient at oxygenating your blood. You will find breathing easier as you clamor up the stairs holding a pile of laundry in one arm and a two-year-old in the other. Running trains your lungs to become stronger, and you will notice a distinct difference as you become more fit.

Keep Your Heart Healthy

As your running improves, so does your cardiovascular system. Your heart becomes more efficient at pushing out more blood per beat and enabling it to beat fewer times per minute. Your blood vessels carrying your blood become stronger and wider, allowing blood to reach your limbs more efficiently. Imagine giving your child a milkshake to drink through a coffee stirrer, then trying again through a wider beverage straw. More volume is able to get through with less suck, which means a happy kid. This is exactly how your blood vessels transform when you run.

The Women's Heart Foundation reports "that 267,000 women die each year from heart attacks . . . six times as many women as

[from] breast cancer. Another 31,837 women die each year of congestive heart failure, representing 62.6 percent of all heart failure deaths." These numbers are staggering and should scare you right into running shoes! According to the Women's Heart Foundation: "One of the safest and most effective ways to reduce your risk and improve your cardiovascular fitness is through aerobic exercise." In fact, simply stepping out the door a few minutes every day is a great start. You can make a difference with your heart health by beginning to move slowly, and then challenging your heart to become stronger in a safe progression of exercise.

Squash Viruses

Hand sanitizer works wonders for a quick wipe-down of lunchroom tables or for cleaning the grocery cart that your baby teethes on, but it is far better to build up your immunity from the inside out. Researchers really aren't sure why running strengthens the immune system; it could be that increased blood flow sends white blood cells and antibodies through more quickly, that the rise in body heat prevents bad bacteria from hanging around, or that running simply blows the airborne viruses right out of the lungs. But whatever the reasons, running improves your ability to fight viral and bacterial infections. The outcome is a healthier, stronger immune system, and once you begin a running regimen, you will likely notice a decrease in the sniffles.

Reduce the Risk of Breast Cancer

Sadly, it's likely that breast cancer has directly affected you or someone you know. Running can be not only preventative but also incredibly helpful to survivors, as it can lower the risk of recurrence. One recent study suggests that women who exercise after fighting breast cancer improve their odds of survival. Running reduces the risk of breast cancer, and many of the contributing factors like obesity, high insulin and estrogen levels, and a compromised immune system disappear with a regular exercise routine. The National Cancer Institute reports: "Exercising four or more hours a week may decrease hormone levels and help lower breast cancer risk. The effect of exercise on breast cancer risk may be greatest in premenopausal women of normal or low weight." Not only that, but the positive mental benefits of running can improve a woman's mood, enhancing the quality of life for someone who is currently fighting breast cancer or is in remission.

Support Your Bones

The National Osteoporosis Foundation (NOF) reports that one in two women is at risk of developing osteoporosis. Osteoporosis most often strikes the bones of your lower body, causing fractures and complete breaks. The NOF recommends thirty minutes of weight-bearing exercise on most days of the week, which can include walking, hiking, playing tennis, or other exercises that are performed while standing Weight-bearing exercises are critical for women as we age, and running is the most efficient at it, strengthening bones in your legs, hips, and lower back. The force of running increases bone mineral density and causes the bone to "reproduce," which strengthens your existing structure.

Develop Sexy Muscle Tone

I once overheard a fit older gentleman explaining how he got such amazingly toned legs. He said: "I ran about 30,000 miles to get my legs to look like this." Fortunately, you won't need to rack up quite so many miles to notice a difference in your legs. In fact, you will notice subtle changes in your muscle tone quickly as your body acclimates to the new movement. From the tip of your toes through your core and even your upper torso, the muscles in your body work together to propel you forward. Primarily you will see benefits in your large muscle groups: your calves and the muscles that make up your thighs, the quadriceps in the front and the hamstring muscles in the back, and, of course, your glute muscles (the muscles that shape your bottom). Running also strengthens your core muscles, allowing you to stand taller and have better balance with an engaged abdomen and backside.

Strengthen Your Joints

Naysayers will tell you that running is bad for your joints and ligaments (those sinewy cords that connect your bones together). Running, they say, will ruin your joints, eventually causing arthritis and pain, but, in fact, a 2008 Stanford study found that there was no difference in occurrences of osteoarthritis between a non-running group and runners. It was participants with a higher BMI (body mass index) who were more likely to be affected by osteoarthritis, and since runners tend to weigh less than the general population, it means they are actually placing less stress on their joints in daily life, decreasing the chances of pain. Joints are only as strong as the muscles that support them, and running will help strengthen the surrounding muscles in the hips, knees, and ankles.

Stabilize Your Gut

No evidence proves that running reduces the number of diapers you'll have to change for your children, but for your own system, running is stool regulation magic. As you adjust to your new running routine, so will your intestinal tract, and you'll start to notice that any moderate constipation problems you may have been experiencing will start to disappear. A 2003 Harvard School of Public Health study found that "women who reported daily physical activity had a lower prevalence of constipation." Running stimulates the nerves and the muscles of the intestinal tract, which will "get things going" for you. In the first few weeks of a running program it may take a bit to learn and understand when your body needs to "go," and there may even be times you are alerted in the middle of a run. But soon enough your body will adapt and you will become a "regular" runner.

Decrease PMS

No matter what you call it—your girlfriend, your bestie, Aunt Flow, or simply your period—running will help you keep premenstrual symptoms in check. Again, researchers aren't sure why (maybe we need more female researchers), but running seems to decrease PMS symptoms. There is nothing better than claiming victory when you beat that crampy, bloated feeling by heading out the door. My husband, who can claim to be a one-man research team, can attest to how running seems to take an edge off my moodiness that time of the month. While men's hormones are rather stable, women's hormones change constantly throughout the month depending on where they are in their menstrual cycle. There may be days that you just don't feel like running, when your breasts are tender and heavy, you are bloated, and nothing feels right. But this just may be the best time to run, as many of the symptoms will be tempered by exercise.

REAL MOMS RUN

I was diagnosed with relapsing-remitting MS when I was twenty-seven years old. So much of my life since diagnosis has centered around what I thought I could not do and my own "excuses" for not doing things. After all, I have a chronic illness, so how can I be expected to be an athlete? When I started running, it was to lose weight, and I never thought I would enjoy it. What I discovered is that I love the discipline of running, if not always the process. I also love the small accomplishments I am able to celebrate. Each mile I have run is one more mile than I thought I ever could run.

—Jennifer, 39, two kids

THE EMOTIONAL BENEFITS

The physical body benefits through running in more ways than we can see—our hearts, lungs, and immune systems all get stronger, and these systems are critical to our well-being, but a clear head is just as important. A healthy mind combined with a healthy body is the win-win we should run toward. The emotional and mental benefits as you begin your running routine will encourage a lifelong habit.

Henry David Thoreau once said: "Methinks that the moment my legs begin to move my thoughts begin to flow." While Thoreau didn't train for a 5K, he did understand that the brain and body function at their best when moving together. Running gives you a chance to create, solve problems, decompress, release stress, and calm an anxious mind.

Meet the Runner's Brain

As you take this running journey and give your body a chance to move, you will soon see how your mind begins to brighten. Body and mind go hand in hand, and the stronger one is the more it encourages the other. The brain works much better when it has sufficient blood flow. As moms we often leave little room in our brain for our own growth, since so much of our mental effort is spent working to manage our family, job, carpools, and deciding which meal is going to land on the table. If you are suddenly faced with a major life change like divorce, illness, death, or a job loss, it's easy for your well-orchestrated schedule to come crashing to the ground. Running gives you your mind back.

Running will be your therapist, your Zen time, and your escape all in one. It can re-energize you, calm you down, or build you up. The brain shrinks with age, and running can help slow that process. Cardiovascular exercise, like walking and running, can stimulate the production of new nerve cells and blood vessels, which helps prevent the brain from shrinking, delaying those "senior moments." Studies have shown that running can increase brain volume, especially in the hippocampus, which affects learning and cognition. You've likely suffered from Mom Brain, an excuse you may use sometimes if you're feeling overwhelmed and forgetful. Let me introduce you to Runner's Brain—when running is a part of your routine, you will feel sharper every day.

Live Better Through Chemistry

Endorphins are chemicals that are released while exercising that interact with the brain and reduce the perception of pain. There are several "feel good" chemicals released during and after you run. You may have heard of a "runner's high," a feeling that comes toward the end of the run that has a positive effect on your outlook the rest of the day. It comes from both the feeling of accomplishment and the chemical reactions going on in your brain.

Neurotransmitters called serotonin and norepinephrine are released during exercise, and they affect your mood and your ability to feel pleasure. Serotonin and norepinephrine are also used to make antidepressants. Running may not cure clinical depression, but the release of chemicals in your brain sure won't make it worse.

Sleep Better

Running is refreshing to a weary body and soul. Heading out for a run after a sleepless night spent with a teething baby sounds counterintuitive, but moving your body will awaken your mind and give you the nudge to get through the day. Running can be the stimulant you need to bridge the gap until you can rest your head again. Pushing the sleepless culprit in a jogging stroller (and of course, she will be sleeping soundly) will refresh your attitude and allow her to sleep. Studies show that exercise shortens the time it takes to fall asleep and improves the quality of sleep, so you will sleep more soundly when it is finally your time for bed.

Boost Confidence

For some reason, as moms, many of us lose the ability to accept a compliment or deem ourselves worthy of praise. A friend compliments you on your fabulous sweater, and instead of standing tall and proudly thanking her, you say: "Oh, this ratty thing? I bought it a Target for three dollars last year." Somewhere in the mom journey it's easy to lose a tiny bit of your own self-worth. You are always doing for others, making sure your family has everything they need before allowing yourself anything. Through your running journey, as you make time for yourself and your fitness improves, your self-confidence will grow too. Your preconceived imperfections will fade as you embrace your healthier form. If you feel strong and beautiful, you will also look strong and beautiful. The brain and the body work together for a healthier whole person through exercise.

RUNNING FOR EVERYONE ELSE

When you choose to exercise, you should do it for yourself and no one else, even though it's sometimes hard to believe that you too are worthy of a little self-indulgence. Just think how much better you would feel if you took even a half-hour alone each day, and how refreshing it could be to rely on and be responsible for only yourself during that time. Consider it a brief recess from kids, laundry, or work—and in the end that time away will renew your outlook and attitude, and you mom abilities improve.

However, if you are struggling with the selfish notion of doing something for yourself, then by all means, use your family, your financial well-being, or a cause that is important to you as justification.

Inspire Your Kids

Today, in the United States, more than 30 percent of our adolescents are overweight or obese. Clearly, we are not only overfeeding our kids, but we are also undermoving them. Children today spend too many sedentary hours in front of the TV, on the computer, and using smartphones. There is even a new syndrome, called iPosture, that comes from too much time with hunched-over shoulders over electronic screens, causing unnecessary pain and poor muscle tone.

You are your children's first role model. How can you expect them to take fitness seriously as a part of their lives if you aren't making it a part of your own? By showing your kids that you care about your body and your health, they will understand the importance and value of exercise. Children understand they need to brush their teeth each night because you instill that as a habit when they are young. Why not do the same with exercise to show that it is necessary for good health? The best way to do that is to lead by example. When you start a running (or any exercise) routine, and make a concerted effort to make the time, your kids will see how important it is. They will quickly learn the value, and understand that movement is not optional—it is part of the family life. As your training becomes habit, your children will become your biggest cheerleaders and will see the difference. This is the first part of raising a healthy child—it starts with you.

You spend a tremendous amount of time driving your children from swim practice to T-ball to lacrosse games—all organized events in which a coach is instructing or a set program is followed. Eventually, they head off to college and away from organized activity. When your child sees you head out the door for a run, he sees you caring for your body on your own without an organized practice or machine. And he will learn that he needs to stay committed to his fitness and health through his whole life. It starts with you.

Your kids often see you as the maid, the driver, the homework helper, and just plain mom. But it is important for them to see you as an individual, with your own goals and desires to improve, enjoy, and enhance your own life. By setting the goal to run a 5K, you are showing your commitment to yourself and that you matter. Your children will begin to see that not everything is about them and that you are an individual with aspirations and desires. It is a healthy realization both physically and mentally. It starts with you.

Save Money

If you are a coupon clipper, or like finding the best possible deals, then running is for you. There is no class fee, no large piece of equipment that needs to be purchased, and no specific place that you have to "belong" to get a run in. Not only that, but running also boasts the highest calorie burn rate per hour of any exercise except cross-country skiing, which requires the investment of equipment and, of course, snow. It may not be totally free—you will need to make an investment in the right shoes and a supportive bra—but dollar for dollar, running is the cheapest form of exercise that you can do. Your bank account will thank you and so will your health insurance.

Give Back to the Community

Whether it is for disaster relief, breast cancer, heart disease, or other charitable causes, 5K fundraisers are an excellent reason to begin running while raising awareness for a cause or an organization that is important to you. Many charitable organizations include training programs and support networks if you agree to raise a certain dollar amount for their cause. For example, the Crohn's and Colitis Foundation of America offers Team Challenge, which is a fundraising team training program that provides wonderful support and benefits for an athlete. Most communities have their own special 5K races. Check community boards at your local running store or online to find one that matches your goals. Running for a charitable cause is always good karma.

REAL MOMS RUN

As a child I was overweight and inactive. I avoided athletic competitions and lagged socially. When I began running, albeit slowly, I discovered a healthy competitive streak. A pivotal moment for me was crossing the finish line at my first race when I heard my name announced over the loudspeaker. I finally realized that I was no longer the "fat kid." I was an athlete. It was a very emotional moment that made me cry. I experienced a positive spillover effect in all areas of my life. Not only had I boosted my physical health, but my appearance and self-confidence improved as well. Most notably, I had tangible proof that if I made a plan to reach a goal, I could do anything I wanted.

—Kris, 53, two kids

CHAPTER 2

The Ingredients of Running

If you choose your dinner recipes based on the minimum number of ingredients and the time it takes to prepare, then you'll love running. It is a minimalist sport, with a small number of ingredients and easy preparation. If you take one part preparation (the right shoes, the right bra), one part determination (really finding the time), and one part perspiration (that's when you really have to get out there and do it), you'll have the perfect recipe for creating a running routine that fits your life. Running can be done anywhere—around your neighborhood, at your child's soccer game, on a trail, or while on vacation. It is as flexible as you are willing to be, but you should know a few important things before getting started.

DRESS THE PART

The right running clothes—shoes, socks, bra, and shorts—can make the difference between a good run and a great run. You don't have to spend a lot of money on these things as long as you follow a few basic guidelines.

Finding the Right Shoe

When your mother gave you advice on picking a spouse, she probably said that you'll likely kiss a lot of frogs before your find your prince and to choose wisely, because it would be the most important decision you ever made. For a runner, shoes are the same. They will become the single most important investment you make, so do your research before buying a running shoe. And just like picking a partner, make sure you try on a lot of shoes before settling on a pair for you.

Once you find the style that works for you, stay true to the shoes and don't be influenced by others or lured by the razzle and dazzle of the latest and greatest. You will know what works for you, and it's important to be loyal—though it's a lot easier to divorce a pair of running shoes than it is a husband.

The Running-Store Experience

If possible, find an independent running retailer where employees are trained to fit athletes of all abilities and sizes. Running stores are a great resource for shoes and gear, a cool place to "talk shop" and learn from more experienced athletes, and may even provide much more, such as organized weekly runs and race information. Don't be intimidated to walk into a running store. They are excited to help you learn about what they already love.

How to Buy Running Shoes

When you first visit a store, tell the salesperson about your running experience (be honest) and your goal to run a 5K. A good employee should be able to pick several options for you based on your size, experience, gait, and foot plant. She should look at your feet without your socks on, watch you walk, and then watch you stand on one foot and then the other. Questions that she should ask are:

- What is your experience?
- How much do you plan to run?
- Where do you plan to run?
- Do you have any prior or current injuries?

If she has only one brand of shoe available, do not feel obligated to buy it. There are other stores. Also be aware that there is no "break-in" period for running shoes. If the shoe doesn't feel good in the store, it won't feel good when you run. Don't be alarmed if the saleswoman fits you in a size of shoe that you only thought worthy of the Jolly Green Giant. Running shoes can be a half size to a size and a half larger than your street shoes. Ask if you can take the shoes outside for a test run, or try them on their treadmill. If you do not live near a running-specific retailer, don't worry. With a little running-shoe know-how, you can find the right shoe for you. Here's how to determine the shoe that will fit you:

- Before going to the store, take an arch test to determine if you need a neutral-cushioned trainer or a motion control (or stability) shoe. This test is easily done by walking with wet feet outside on dry pavement. Walk naturally in a straight line, then turn around and evaluate your arch type.

  » **Normal arch:** If your wet footprint shows your toes, the ball of your foot, and about half your arch (the outside half) before showing your entire heel, your arch is normal. This type of footprint indicates that your foot would be best suited for a neutral-cushioned shoe.

  » **Flatfoot:** If your entire footprint is filled in on the concrete, then you are flatfooted or an overpronator, which means your foot has more inward movement when you step. Look for a shoe with more structure, called a stability shoe or a motion control shoe. These shoes offer various levels of support and are also helpful for overweight runners.

  » **High arch:** If your wet footprint shows just your toes, the ball and heel of your foot, and a little bit of the outside of your foot, then you have a high arch, or supinate, meaning your foot rolls outward. This foot type does best in a neutral-cushioned trainer.

- Find several pairs in your size and try on each, checking for adequate space in the front. The front of the shoe is called the toe box, and you should try to get the equivalent of a thumb's width there (press your thumb down horizontally between your toes and the end of the shoe). Keep in mind that your feet swell as the day goes on, so that can also affect your shoe size. If you are pregnant or postnatal, your foot size can also be larger than normal.

- Check the back of the shoe, called the heel box, for movement. You should be able to slide a finger inside the shoe along your inside (medial) ankle bone. Too much and you will roll your ankle, too little and you will be blistered in no time.
- Consider a stability shoe if you are overweight. The extra structure can save your joints until they acclimate to running.
- Now take all the shoes for a test drive. Ask to take them outside; if the store doesn't permit it, jog around a few of the store aisles. Remember: They must feel good in the store.

Running shoes generally last for about 300 to 500 miles of running depending on your weight and the type of surface you run on. Usually your joints will tell you when you need to replace your shoes, but if you are unsure, take them into a running store to be evaluated. If you have had a pair of shoes for several years with little wear, it still may be time to invest in a new pair. The materials used for running shoes lose their cushiness after time. Many runners buy two pairs and rotate them, ensuring that they will have the same model for a longer period. Once you find a pair you like, there is no reason to change. Don't be tempted by color, design, or the latest shoe being promoted. Defer to fit and feel, and trust your gut.

Socks

Your shoes are only as good as the socks you put in them. Since these are your cushions to the concrete, it is smart to pay attention and choose well. With all your clothes, from the socks to your top, keep in mind this simple motto for the running world: "Cotton Is Rotten." Cotton socks can bunch up, hold sweat, and cause blisters to form, while running socks are generally made of synthetic, breathable blend fabrics, which can contain smaller amounts of cotton or wool that wick moisture away from your feet and minimize friction. There are several styles of running socks, so it may take you a few runs to sort out your preference for height and thickness. Some running socks even have a left foot-right foot designation with the toe of the sock slanted as from big toe to small. Don't buy the six-pair package until you're sure what works for you. Some runners prefer thin, barely there socks and others prefer thicker, more cushioned socks, and your preference may even change depending on the season.

Running Bras

Minimizing your breast movement can greatly affect your running experience. Too much bounce and you will be uncomfortable and in pain, or if you're too restricted and compressed, your pain may be even worse. Whether you're a AA or a DDDD, any woman can experience breast pain when she runs, so a well-fitted bra will minimize discomfort.

Dr. Joanna Scurr, a researcher at the University of Portsmouth in the United Kingdom, studies the biomechanics of the breast while running and has determined that the breast moves in nearly every direction while a woman runs, no matter the cup size. So it is logical that a supportive bra would reduce the amount of movement, enabling a more comfortable run. Running can cause breasts to sag if your bra is not supportive, and with so many other things already causing saggy breasts (genetics, age, and those adorable kids you birthed and fed), why add another to the list? Look for the following qualities when shopping for bras:

- **High MCR (motion control rating) bras:** Most exercise bras are rated for the amount of exercise bounce they can endure. For example, a low MCR rating would be suitable for yoga or Pilates, but when running you want to keep the bounce to a minimum, no matter what your size, so opt for a high MCR rating.
- **Bras that encapsulate each breast in a separate chamber:** This will reduce bounce and is recommended for B cups and larger. If you are medium

to large breasted, then avoid compression-type bras that mush your breasts together.

- **Bras that come in cup and band sizes:** Look for your bra size versus just small, medium, or large, as these types of bra are designed to fit your chest size more precisely.
- **Comfort:** Try on several different styles to determine what is most comfortable for you. Check seams, hooks, and straps, and feel for areas that might dig into your shoulder, at your cleavage, or around your torso.
- **Moisture wicking:** Fabrics like Coolmax or Dri-FIT pull moisture away from your body, reducing chafing.

Most importantly, find the style that works for you. Experiment with many different styles: racerback, traditional, pullover, or clasped. Keep in mind that a running bra is not designed for all-day comfort and may feel restrictive if you wear it too long. However, once again, if it isn't comfortable in the store, it will be even worse on your run.

If you haven't been sized in a while, get properly fitted. Most of us spend our life in a misfit bra, keeping the same size from graduation through our pregnancies without ever being properly fit by a specialist. Now is a good time to make sure you've got the right size. It is especially important to be fit properly if you are pregnant or breastfeeding. While you don't need a breastfeeding bra, you do need to pay special attention to the restriction that a running bra places on your breasts or you could end up compressing your milk ducts, causing mastitis.

Take a "test drive" to make sure the bra works for you: jump up and down, and swing your arms to determine if there is any area that is bothersome. It should feel comfortable on the first hook. Bras loosen up and lose their elasticity as they age, so you will need the extra hooks for the life of the bra. Whatever you choose, you should be able to get a year out of your bra if you don't put it in the dryer. Other than your shoes, this will be your most important running purchase, so take the time to make the right decision.

Running Clothes

The most important factor in running clothes is comfort. You don't need to spend money on a top brand or the latest style. Simply wear what is comfortable for you. It is easy to get caught up in the technical details of running gear and feel like you *need* to have a $125 jacket or a $75 technical shirt. Companies like Jockey make affordable active wear for the everyday athlete that can be purchased at department stores everywhere or easily online. (You can find more specific recommendations for clothing, shoes, and more on the resources page of my website, *www.RunLikeaMother.com*.) Here are a few tips when making your clothing selection:

- Remember: Cotton is Rotten. Choose synthetic fabrics or blends that pull moisture away from your body, keeping you cool in the summer and dry in the winter. Look for items that say Coolmax or Dri-FII on the label, as these fabrics are engineered for performance.
- Comfort is key. Binding, tight, restrictive clothing will cause redness, chafing, and blisters. If you find you chafe regardless of the clothing item, try using BodyGlide or other sports lubricant that can be found at your local running store. If you are overweight, consider the length of the shorts and the material, because loose clothing or not enough fabric can also cause painful chafing between your legs. Compression-style shorts work well under your running shorts to prevent chafing.
- If you are between seasons or running in the winter, dress in layers so that you can peel as you get warm. Avoid vests that you can't tie around your waist when the temperature rises. A good rule of thumb is to dress as if it is twenty degrees warmer than what the real temperature is: If it is 60°F outside,

dress for 80°F weather. Always bring an additional layer to throw on after you run so that you stay warm until you get the sweaty clothes off.

- Buy dollar store stretchy gloves, the kind that will fit both your four-year-old and your husband. I buy them in large quantities in different styles at the beginning of winter, and I don't worry if one is misplaced. I love it when my husband dons a glitter snowflake glove on one hand and a striped one on the other to shovel snow.

- A running cap will protect you from the elements and keep your face safe from the sun. Your son's baseball cap will work, but there are running-specific caps that have terry cloth headbands built in to keep your eyes free of sweat. Look for a cap that has the nifty keyhole opening in back; it is a great way to keep your ponytail in check. Running caps are machine washable too.

- Dress to be seen. If you spend most of your time sharing your running route with cars, then it is imperative to dress in bright clothes. Consider clothing with reflective properties if you run at dawn, dusk, or in the dark. Also consider a headlamp that has a bright white light in front and a blinking red light in the back. You will see the road better in front of you and be seen by traffic in both directions.

A Digital Watch with Chronograph Option

You can run without a watch, with your great-grandmother's analog, or with a smartphone, however a valuable inexpensive investment would be a simple digital watch. Most have a chronograph option, or the ability to time your runs. A simple digital watch that provides cumulative time and also allows you to record laps so that you time your run/walk intervals is adequate. Many are now available in bright colors and also look great in daily life. A digital watch with a timer (chronograph) option can be purchased for as little as $25 at major retailers.

Running Wish List Items

Your love of running will open up a whole new list of must-haves in your wardrobe. These are not accessories that you need to make you faster, though they will motivate you with bling and technology:

1. **Elastic stash belt:** There are many manufacturers that make belts with little pouches that will hold keys or a phone if you need to carry one while you run. They fit the contour of your body and keep items from jiggling while you run. They can be a fun fashion statement with leopard print and razzle-dazzle or sleek and stealth in black.
2. **Headband:** Performance headbands are fun and functional. They come in thousands of patterns and thicknesses and really allow your style to show in the sweatiest of times, and best of all, they don't slip while running.
3. **Multifunction digital watch:** There are options available that give directions, register heart rate, predict the weather, and tell you when you should start and stop running. Some also allow your family to see exactly where you are running using GPS or smartphone technology, and even allow you to upload to the computer and analyze data.

RUNNING DECONSTRUCTED

Now that you know how to look the part, it's important to understand how to make your body move. There are simple techniques that will help you move forward more efficiently, and as you become comfortable with your running, these movements can strengthen your gait and will make you more efficient. The beauty of running is that you shouldn't have to think about it too much. (If you want more analysis, I suggest you try golf.) Let's deconstruct some of the movements to make sure your form is helping you stay comfortable and safe.

Hit Your Stride

As much as you would like to imagine yourself running with the elongated stride of a graceful gazelle, as a new runner, it is important to let your feet land directly beneath you and not try to force a longer stride, because forcing it will put unnatural force on your joints and put you in an unsafe situation. As you become stronger and more experienced, your body may naturally adapt to a slightly longer stride length, but for now, attempting to morph your stride into something it is not is the quickest way to injury.

Sports scientist, Olympic athlete, and coach, Jack Daniels, PhD, has determined that runners are most efficient and less prone to injury when the stride rate is 180 steps per minute (each foot strike counting as one). This higher cadence allows you to spend less time suspended in the air, and your feet will enjoy a softer landing, minimizing injury. During the first weeks of training, count your stride rate for 1 minute and assess your cadence. While your cadence will vary a bit with speed and terrain, striving for 180 steps per minute is good practice. As you progress in the program you can test and reassess periodically to improve your turnover.

Stand Tall

Maintaining good posture while you run maximizes the amount of air you take in and engages your core, allowing you to get the most out of your midsection. Think about running tall from your hips to your shoulders without becoming too rigid; your shoulders do not need to be back like a soldier, but rather loose with a slight forward roll.

Relax Your Face

Right now I want you to smile. I'm not talking about a forced "cheese" smile, but rather a soft, natural smile. Now drop your mouth open, and relax your muscles. A loose, open jaw will relax the muscles of your face. Running with your mouth open makes it easier to breathe. If you run with a clenched jaw, those tensed muscles in your mouth will radiate down your neck and into the rest of your body. Keep your mouth loose and your body will follow.

Keep Your Head Up

While your face is relaxed, your head should be straight so that your line of sight is about eight to fifteen feet in front of you. Keeping your head in this forward, neutral position will be most comfortable and allow you to see and react to any terrain changes. If you are running on a treadmill, keep your sight focused forward or on the console, as looking down can set you off balance.

Swing Your Arms

Pretend for a moment that you have your daughter's ballet tutu around your waist. Now swing your arms forward and back at a 90-degree angle. Your arms should swing nicely above the tutu as they go back with your hand almost touching at hip (tutu) level. As they move forward, your shoulders should be the only joint moving as your elbows stay bent at 90 degrees. When your arms come forward, your hands should not cross your midline, nor should they venture above the shoulder. Most of your upper body should be relaxed with the arms swinging forward, not twisting or turning, as that will use excess energy and throw you off balance.

Lean Forward

A little bit of a forward lean will help propel your forward movement. Stand tall and lean just a little bit from the ankles and soften the hips. Don't bend at the waist or stick your bottom out, just lean from the ankles and that will be enough to get you in the right position for running.

Keep Your Hands Loose

Run as if you are holding a thin potato chip between your thumb and your first finger—not a fat tortilla chip, but the most delicate of chips. This is how relaxed and loose your hands should be while running. Your palms should be facing inward with thumbs up. Clenching your fists as you run will cause stress all the way up the arm and into the shoulder and across the chest, which will throw off your stride.

Just Breathe

Like that Faith Hill song says: "Just breathe." You have been doing it for years and never given it a second thought. If you start thinking about your breathing, you might end up hyperventilating. There are hundreds of theories determining how an athlete should breathe while running: inhale for three steps, exhale for two; in through the nose, out through the mouth; and it goes on from there. When it comes to breathing, just don't run faster than you can breathe. Keeping your jaw loose and your mouth open provides you with lots of options: nose breathing, mouth breathing, or a combination of the two. Determining what is comfortable comes when you aren't aware of how you are getting your breath.

If you are new to exercise, this is an important lesson. The training program in Part 2 of this book is geared toward conversation pace, meaning that you should be able to have a nice conversation while you run and be able to answer questions in short sentences, not in breathless affirmations or frantic head bobs. If you can talk, you can breathe. And if you run alone, a good test is trying to sing a show tune or your favorite children's song. As the weeks progress in training, you will become more efficient and the pace will pick up with the same amount of effort. If you find yourself winded, struggling for air, or with a side stitch, slow down, and your breath will recover.

WHERE IN THE WORLD DO I RUN?

You know what to wear and how to move your body, but now where should this new exercise happen? The options are limitless. Out your front door, around the track, on the treadmill, or at a trail, running can be done anywhere in the world provided you understand the rules of the road, run aware of your surroundings, and run defensively. The two most important things to think about when choosing where to run are surface and safety.

The best way to deal with oncoming traffic, the approach of a sketchy looking individual, or a stray dog is to practice mindful running. Mindful running means to run in the moment, being aware of not only your body but where you are and who is around you. As you begin to run, you have many choices where to exercise outside: concrete, asphalt, trail, or track. There are pros and cons to each, and as you become accustomed to running you will find your own preference.

Road Runners

Most of us live in areas that have hard running surfaces, such as sidewalks and roads that are made of concrete and asphalt. Sidewalks are the safest place to run, and in most states legally you have to use the sidewalk when running if there is one available on your route. The downside of the sidewalk is the hardness of concrete and the potential that poorly maintained walks can have lifted edges or crevices that pose tripping hazards. Asphalt provides a better cushion, which can help dampen your foot strike and cause less stress to your body. If you choose to run on the road, there are several rules you should follow to ensure your own safety:

- Always run against traffic when sharing the road. This means that you should be running on the left side of the road and facing oncoming cars. You want to see the car so you can react if the driver doesn't see you.
- Make eye contact with drivers as they approach you. Just because they are driving in a straight line doesn't mean they see you. Try to look at their eyes, and a friendly wave will alert them to your presence.
- Wear bright clothing when running on the road, especially in areas that aren't well lit.
- If an oncoming car is closer than you feel is comfortable, try sticking your hand out to your side as the car approaches, ensuring you have a comfortable amount of room to run.
- When approaching a blind corner, cross the road in a place where there is good visibility of traffic in both directions ahead of the corner, and then return as soon as conditions are safe.
- Be aware that if you are running in the road with snow banks that a car has limited room to move away from you. Consider the sidewalk or finding an area to run that is less affected, such as a treadmill or the track at your local high school.

Trailblazers

If you are lucky enough to live in an area that has trails or dirt roads, try to do most of your running on them. Trails not only provide a more cushioned surface, but they are also free from cars and congestion, and usually offer (much needed) peace and quiet. Some trails have mile markers, though you should always be mindful of your surroundings and run with a partner or tell someone at home where you are going and when you will be back. Trails and dirt roads provide a wonderful respite from traffic; however, this doesn't mean you should let down your guard—always be aware of the path directly beneath and in front of you. If you are a new runner, seek trails that are wide dirt, cinder path, parkways, or rail trails. These trails offer a softer surface and are typically less technical to navigate.

Track Stars

A high-school or community track is the flattest, safest, softest manmade surface to run on. Tracks, whether they are made of the old-school cinder or the newer rubberized surface, are measured out in either 400-yard or 400-meter ovals, which makes keeping track of mileage simple. Four laps on the inside lane is usually equivalent to a mile. Tracks are a great meeting place for moms, because if the facility permits, the kids can play on the inside field while you run around them. Stagger a few moms running around the track and the children are never farther than a quick sprint away. Preschool and grade-school children who can follow the rules of the track may even join in and run a few laps too. The downside to track running is that feeling that you're a mouse on an exercise wheel: round and round, over and over the same scenery. If you struggle with quitting before a workout is over, running on a track can be a challenge, as you are never too far away from the start. There are just a few things to remember when running on a track:

- Check to see if there are posted hours that the public is allowed to run. Some schools do not permit you to run while it is in session; others allow it but want you to check in at the main office.
- Look to see if there is a sign posted indicating the direction you are to run. Many tracks rotate directions depending on the day of the week, though most typically run counterclockwise.
- Run in the correct lane. The inside lane is reserved for the fastest person on the track at the moment. If no one is there, have at it, otherwise concede to the fastest runner even if you were there first.
- Pass on the outside of the runner. If you are running counterclockwise that is the right; running clockwise would be on the left.

Treading Lightly

Running outside is wonderful though not always possible. Inclement weather, lack of child care, and unsafe outside light can all be reasons to keep it inside. The treadmill can be a blessing to any mom that does not have the ability to run outside. Many runners actually prefer treadmill running and feel more comfortable and confident in a controlled environment because it allows the flexibility of running a distance or time without determining if a route is long enough, and it affords the ability to stop when necessary. Treadmills also offer a shock-absorbing, rubberized surface and the ability to control time, pace, and elevation, and some even calculate heart rate and calorie burn. Treadmills can be found at gyms, health clubs, YMCAs, and hotels, and though the type of instrument panel varies, they all do the same thing: They let you run. Before stepping onto a treadmill, familiarize yourself with the following:

- All treadmills have an emergency shutoff pulley or button to immediately stop the tread from moving. Make sure you know where it is.
- Take a good look at the display panel before starting the treadmill. Opt for the manual mode if unfamiliar with the treadmill, as this will allow you to control the speed and elevation.
- Always start with a walking pace on an unfamiliar treadmill. By walking first you can familiarize yourself with the belt speed and adjust to how it feels.
- Setting the elevation to 1 percent more closely replicates running outside. If you are just getting started it is fine to keep the treadmill at 0 percent elevation, and then gradually work your way up and experiment with different elevations.
- Do not change your running style while on the treadmill. Set the pace so that you can run at your normal gait. If you increase the pace or incline so much that you have to change the way you move, you will open the door to injury.

Your body gets a slightly different workout on the treadmill, as the "ground" is moving underneath you. Varying the incline will help compensate for some of the loss of range through your gait cycle. Many treadmills have programmed routes that will change the grade automatically so that you can't cheat the hills. All of the training programs in Chapter 4 can be done easily on the treadmill; simply adjust the speed between the walks and runs, and use the treadmill clock to time your intervals.

See Mom Groove

Music can be a great motivator while running. If you choose to wear a headset, remember to keep the volume low or one earplug out so that you can hear the sounds of approaching vehicles, dogs, or people. While everyone's taste in music is different, here are just a few songs that might make you move:

1. Gym Class Heroes, "Fighter"
2. Kanye West, "Stronger"
3. Rob Base and DJ E-Z Rock, "It Takes Two"
4. Wreckx-n-Effect, "Rump Shaker"
5. U2, "Beautiful Day"
6. Survivor, "Eye of the Tiger"
7. Eminem, "Lose Yourself"
8. Black Eyed Peas, "Let's Get It Started"
9. Shakira, "Waka Waka"
10. Bill Conti, "Gonna Fly Now"
11. Bruce Springsteen, "Born to Run"

Techno-Running

In today's world of apps, smartphones, and GPS devices, it is easy to get wrapped up in gear and forget what running is all about. Though many devices and programs promote running by giving you audible cues to slow down, pick up the pace, walk, or finish the workout, keep in mind that running is a pure sport and too much of an electronic thing can alter your heart rate (up-tempo songs may make you run too fast), cause you to change your pace at the wrong time, or distract you from the road and sounds around you. Rely on yourself, listen to your body, and enjoy the run.

TIME MANAGEMENT

The biggest challenge as a mom is finding the time, and when it is finally available, finding the mojo to run. The hardest part of beginning a running program is understanding that to find time, you have to create it. With our children's activities we spend a tremendous amount of effort making sure they get to practice or rehearsal on time and stay for the entire session. Your exercise needs should be addressed in the same fashion.

The Centers for Disease Control and Prevention (CDC) advises that adults should get 150 minutes of moderate to vigorous exercise a week. That is five days of 30 minutes of exercise, and that is our U.S. government speaking. The benefits of exercise begin to reveal themselves at 150 minutes of movement. If you need to break it into smaller chunks over six days or larger chunks over three days, fitting the time in however you can counts. If only the U.S. government agenda could find a twenty-fifth hour in a mom's day so we could fit it all in.

Create a Partner Program

If you have a partner at home, start there. Schedule time three days a week during which you can watch the children for forty-five minutes and vice versa. You might have to get creative with time at first, but scheduling it in for both of you, back to back, will aid in compliance. Having a running partner, even when you do it separately, can be a great bonding experience, as you encourage and support each other's efforts.

Just make sure to alternate who goes first each time, so that if your child tends to become needy during the second hour, it doesn't always fall on the same parent. You can also try switching days: you get Monday, he gets Tuesday. In this case, the easiest time to exercise is the early morning before the house wakes up, but figure out what works best for you and go with it.

Find a Running Group

When I first began running, I joined a women's running "co-op" through our local park district called the Racy Ladies. Several days a week we would meet with our children in tow at the local recreation center. The kids would get to play in the gym, and we would rotate which moms would run and which would babysit. Because the run-sitter rotation changed, we got to run and meet with different moms each week. Many years and several moves later, this running group remains a fond memory for my girls and me. The group collectively paid the rental of the recreation center gym for about an hour and half, so the cost to run was minimal. More importantly, knowing that I always had running buddies to rely on for support was always a great motivator.

Many YMCAs and gyms provide their own childcare while you exercise, and might already have running programs in place. Confirm first whether they let you leave to run outside before committing, though many also have indoor tracks. You can also check your local running store because they often have groups available that fit your schedule or a bulletin board with listings of programs and events.

If there isn't a recreation center or you don't have the resources to join a group, consider swapping with a friend who has small children. Schedule your swapped workouts like you would any other weekly commitment. Get it on the calendar. It could be at a home, or consider meeting up at a park and taking turns running around the park while the kids play. By setting a schedule, your children will become accustomed to the routine and will look forward to your running time and their playdate. When my children were babies, I never made a lunch date or social outing unless it involved running or walking. If I needed a sitter, to meet with someone socially or for work, I always requested a "running" lunch or meeting. If that person didn't run, then I encouraged them to walk. Try killing the "ladies' lunch" and instituting the "women's run." It's cheaper and the conversation is just as engaging.

If you are still finding it difficult to slip away for an hour a few days a week, try breaking up your run up into smaller bites of time. You will benefit just as much from twenty minutes in the morning and another twenty minutes later. Exercise counts whenever and however you get it in. Keep a small bag of running clothes in your car; you never know when there might be a time between carpools and appointments to squeeze in a run. The thrill of finding that precious moment to squeeze in a quick run can be as exhilarating as the run itself. A bonus run in a hectic day will feel like stolen time.

Dawn of the Runner

One way to fit in a quick run is to head out the door very early in the morning. You may not always be able to control where your day takes you, but you can usually control when it starts. Getting it done before everyone wakes up is a wonderful way to start the day. It may take a few weeks for your body to adjust and to master sneaking out of the house quietly. Try laying your clothes out the night before outside your room so that you aren't disturbing your sleeping family.

If you decide that this is your time to run, it's important that you wear reflective gear and bright-colored clothing. It is important to be seen and for you to see where you're going. If you are running when it is dark out or not well lit, a runner's headlamp is a great way to light the way while keeping your hands free.

When you run at night or in the predawn hours, you should remember three simple rules: Tell, Vary, and Carry.

Tell someone where you are running and when you will be home.

Vary your route. You might think your loved ones know your route because you run it three times a week, but assume that your family doesn't and that a creepy person might.

Carry ID. It is smart to always have identification with you when you run. No need to carry a purse; it is as simple as photocopying your ID and sticking it in your pocket or writing your name and number on the inside of a shirt. You can even buy nifty runner-friendly ID bands or shoe charms.

A Woman's Best Friend

Most dogs that approach you, whether you are running or not, simply want to greet you. It is important to familiarize yourself with the dogs on your route and change your run if there is a dog that is threatening. If you are running and encounter a loose dog that appears aggressive and is headed in your direction, the Humane Society provides these tips to protect yourself:

1. Resist the impulse to scream and run away.
2. Remain motionless, hands at your sides, and avoid eye contact with the dog.
3. Once the dog loses interest in you, slowly back away until he is out of sight.
4. If the dog does attack, "feed" him your jacket or anything that you can put between yourself and the dog.
5. If you fall or are knocked to the ground, curl into a ball with your hands over your ears and remain motionless. Try not to scream or roll around.

Finding the Mojo

So you finally have the time—your clothes are on, your shoes are laced, the kids are with a friend—and suddenly you just want to curl up in a ball on the couch with a bowl of popcorn and a book. Remind yourself why you have set aside this time, why it is important, and how much better you will feel once you step out the door.

The most difficult struggle as a mom trying to adhere to a running or any exercise program is carving out the time on a regular basis and setting a family schedule that includes your running time. But when you do, the opportunities are endless, because running can be done almost anywhere and at any time. It is hard to have an excuse not to run. Although the couch may seem inviting after a difficult day, the run will be more rewarding. Remember to always be aware of your surroundings; share the road, the trail, or the track with respect for all those that approach; and defend your space when necessary.

REAL MOMS RUN

My daughter and I went through some pretty tough times between her thirteenth and eighteenth year. She took our family on a hard, chaotic journey. During that time, I ran to keep my strength and sanity. She is now twenty-two. She and I ran our first 5K together this year in May. It was the most wonderful Mother's Day present I ever received. She and I have gone on to do several more races together this year. I feel so lucky to be able to run with my daughter; it's enough inspiration to keep me running as long as I'm able.

—Anne, 56, two kids

CHAPTER 3

Being Woman

Marilyn Monroe once said, "I don't mind living in a man's world as long as I can be a woman in it." Even with all the stages and changes in a woman's life, I don't think many of us would change who we are. We menstruate, we have babies, we lactate, and then we shut it all down in a dramatic fashion called menopause. Even if you have never given birth, your body was designed around the ability to do so, and the hormones ebb and flow through the months and years just the same. Hormone levels affect your appetite, energy, moods, how your jeans fit, and whether you are a B cup one day and a D the next. Through all these fluctuations, running can be the great smoothing factor, helping to keep the hills from being mountains and the valleys from being canyons. Your running routine might change through the stages of your life, however the benefits will always be rewarding and sometimes lifesaving. As you run through the stages of life, you will learn how running can help you, when you might need to adjust your pace, and when running just might be the adjustment you need to improve your outlook and well-being.

RUNNING AND MENSTRUATION

Remember when you first got your period and it seemed like life as you knew it was over? How were you going to participate in gym class? Were you ever going to be able to wear a swimsuit again?

Then as the months turned into years, your period became a part of your life routine.

It is important for you to know that you can run during all phases of your menstrual cycle. There will be some days when you may not feel like heading out to run and then run surprisingly faster than normal. Then on other days you will want to run but will struggle to keep a pace, feeling labored and heavy. Many women aren't fazed by their cyclical changes and never notice a difference while running, while others will be affected by the slightest hormone fluctuation. Ultimately, running's benefits will help smooth the effects of your cycle and aid in diminishing menstrual symptoms that bother you.

From the first day of your menstrual cycle (the day your period starts) and through the first two weeks, your hormone levels are at their lowest. Typically, this is when you will feel the most invincible as a runner: Your pace will be faster, your energy will be higher, and your outlook will be most positive. Running during your period may be inconvenient at first, but soon enough you will be skilled at timing your runs around your blood flow. If your 5K race coincides with your period, a small fanny pack can hold supplies or you can tape a tampon to the back of your race bib.

During the next two weeks (days 14 through 28 of your cycle), your body may start to feel more sluggish as the increase of hormones can begin to weigh you down. During this time, you could experience a higher than normal heart rate, more labored breathing, and some fluid retention, which can affect your running economy. The week before your period (or about days 20 to 28 of your cycle) when premenstrual syndrome (or PMS) strikes, sometimes the last thing you may feel like doing is running, and yet that is when you should nudge yourself to run. Mentally, it will help you to get out of a PMS funk and refresh your attitude.

About 85 percent of menstruating women have at least one PMS symptom according to the American Congress of Obstetricians and Gynecologists (ACOG). Even if you don't suffer from extreme symptoms, like serious cramps or migraines, it is common to experience general malaise, fatigue, moodiness, bloating, cramps, breast tenderness, and headaches. Any of these symptoms can affect how you interact with people. Your kids, your partner, and your running buddies probably know when to tiptoe around you during this "delicate" time, but it can also affect if and when you get out for a run. Studies are mixed on whether running really alleviates PMS, but most women I know say it helps tremendously. Even if it just takes your mind off the symptoms, that seems like a good enough reason to head out the door.

It may take a few cycles to understand how your period affects your running and some time to adjust to your blood flow and timing of your runs. For this reason, I love darker-colored running shorts and small waist packs.

REAL MOMS RUN

My favorite running buddy is my daughter. She inspires me, she understands me, she entertains me. She also encourages me to keep running even when I'm not prepared.

—Kris, 53, two kids

RUNNING AND PREGNANCY

Running and pregnancy can be a complementary combination, and most doctors will encourage you to maintain a pre-pregnancy fitness routine that adjusts in intensity as the months advance. Running can reduce pregnancy symptoms, such as nausea, fatigue, leg cramps, constipation, and backaches, and can also help maintain muscle tone, increase energy, regulate necessary weight gain, decrease labor time, and ease delivery. As long as you don't have any other complications, most doctors would recommend exercising gently and adjusting your intensity as your pregnancy progresses.

Exercise is part of the preparatory phase of nurturing our baby: creating a healthy womb and then preparing our bodies for the life we are about to lead. Although the ACOG approves of continuing your running routine under the guidance of your physician if you have already been running, pregnancy is not the time to start a new training program. There are thousands of 5K training programs out there, but none are specific to training while pregnant, and for good reason. If you have not run prior to pregnancy, you might not possess the ability to recognize critical warning signals that your body could send indicating that something is wrong. When you're pregnant, you should always consult your doctor about the best exercise and training methods. If you're a non-runner, I would recommend the Creeping Program in this book, where you will train by walking, because it will be the easiest to begin and maintain throughout your pregnancy. The Creeping Program can be safely used throughout your pregnancy as long as your doctor agrees.

Many physical changes during pregnancy will affect how comfortable running will be for you. Some women stop during the first trimester, while others practically run through the doors of the labor and delivery floor at the hospital. There are women who have run marathons and delivered the next day, naming their babies Miles, for the time they shared on the road. Maintaining good communication with your doctor on any issues that arise is important and will help you determine if and when it is advisable to stop. Contrary to past conceptions, there are no fetal or maternal health issues with regular exercise during an uncomplicated pregnancy. Again and again, studies show that a pregnant woman who maintains a fitness regimen fairs better through the pregnancy, delivery, and into recovery.

Benefits of Maintaining an Exercise Program Through Pregnancy

- Better sleep
- Lower chance of unhealthy weight gain
- Improved mood and energy
- Better maintenance of pre-pregnancy muscle tone
- Reduction of constipation and bloating
- Lower chance of gestational diabetes and preeclampsia
- Faster labor and delivery than a sedentary woman
- Quicker return to fitness post-pregnancy

Rate of Perceived Exertion

The best advice for running while pregnant (or at any time) is to listen to your body, paying attention to how you feel during and about two hours after exercise. If you are comfortable while running, then you are exercising at a safe pace. If after a run you are unable to work and take care of your children or are completely wiped out, then it is too much. Running while pregnant should be at a pace that will leave you energized.

The ACOG doesn't recommend a certain pace or heart rate. Instead, it utilizes the Borg Scale of rate of perceived exertion (RPE), which qualifies how you feel while exercising. The modified version of the scale uses numbers from zero to ten to rank your level of breathing. These ratings are very subjective based on how you are feeling.

MODIFIED BORG SCALE OF RATE OF PERCEIVED EXERTION

Rating	Description
0	Nothing at all
1	Very light
2	Fairly light
3	Moderate
4	Somewhat hard
5	Hard
6	
7	Very hard
8	
9	
10	Very, very hard (maximal)

While pregnant and running, the ACOG recommends that you stay between levels three and five, which is a conversation pace. You will begin to lose the ability to talk easily when you are higher than five on the scale. If you can sing a song or talk in complete sentences, you are running at a moderate pace. A newer runner should try to stay around three, while an experienced runner might venture closer to five. The most important thing is to listen to your body. When you feel uncomfortable or unsafe, discontinue the exercise. Remember that pregnancies are as different as the children we produce. Every woman experiences different things, and if you've had more than one child, you know that even the same woman can experience different things during pregnancies. Running may be tolerable for some pregnancies and not others, so make sure you are very mindful of the warning sign so you can stay healthy and safe.

Warning Signs to Terminate Exercise While Pregnant
- Vaginal bleeding
- Shortness of breath prior to exercise
- Dizziness
- Headache
- Chest pain
- Muscle weakness
- Abnormal calf pain or swelling
- Preterm labor
- Decreased fetal movement
- Amniotic fluid leakage

Ways to Keep Your Cool While Pregnant and Exercising
1. Avoid the heat of the day. Run early in the morning or later in the evening, or opt for the treadmill in a climate-controlled facility.
2. Increase fluid intake to replace what you lose during exercise.
3. Pay attention to overheating warnings—nausea, faintness, feeling very hot, and profuse sweating.

Body Changes

Women can gain up to two pounds per breast during pregnancy, which can cause discomfort and stress on the shoulders and back. If this is a problem for you, try doubling up on bras—wearing one racerback and one traditional strapped bra works well. Large-breasted pregnant women may prefer to move to an exercise with less impact such as the elliptical or even water running.

Your pregnant belly is the biggest physical limiter (and rightfully so) to running. The extra weight and size changes your center of gravity and can make balance difficult. If you are experiencing balance issues, take your running to a track or area that is flat to reduce the risk of falling. Some women find running with a pregnancy belt helps them feel more stable. The belt, which is secured under your growing belly, gives added support to the front side and lower back. Pregnancy support belts can be purchased at maternity stores and come in sizes that also have adjustments to accommodate your ever-changing body.

See Mom Run Baby Names

1. Bolt
2. Cadence
3. Dash
4. Chase
5. Quick
6. Walker
7. Pace
8. Lane
9. Miles
10. Brooks

Keep in mind that if you are not comfortable running when pregnant that there are many ways to exercise that are lower impact such as water exercise, stationary bikes, or elliptical machines. Your body is working very hard to create a baby and some days it may signal that rest is best, but generally walking for 30 minutes a day can be enough to promote wellness during pregnancy. Revise your plans according to your growing size, and don't punish yourself for not being able to exercise the way you used to. Applaud yourself for getting out and moving. Even if you need to discontinue running, or exercise altogether, nine months passes quickly, and it's easy to keep your eye on the prize: a healthy labor, delivery, and bundle of joy.

POSTPARTUM RUNNING

Whether it is your first or your fourth baby, making new family adjustments, and dealing with sleep deprivation, takes maternal time management to a whole new level of selflessness. You have created a being and that being needs you. In the first few weeks as you adjust to this crazy, wonderful life called motherhood, your mind and body need to adapt and heal. It took nine months of total body transformation on your part to produce a tiny miracle, and you shouldn't expect to lace up and head out too quickly. You have experienced many physiological changes, and your body can take up to one year to return to normal.

Always consult your doctor before you return to exercise. If your pregnancy and delivery were uncomplicated, then she may let you determine when you are ready to run, but Cesarean sections and episiotomies may slow your return to exercise, as your body should concentrate its energy on healing these wounds. To ease back into running, try to take a 10- to 15-minute walk once or twice a day outside just to clear your mind and move your body a bit.

Your body will need time to return to its pre-pregnancy condition, and even then you may find that you have a "new" you. Your hips that widened to accommodate your pregnancy may remain wider and your abdomen may be a little softened, the skin not as taut. There is nothing like extra skin to remind you that you birthed those babes. Your shoe size may get bigger and your bra size smaller, but these are all changes that come with pregnancy and motherhood, and they are things you will have to adjust to when restarting your running routine.

Returning to the Road

Even if your doctor gives you clearance and you begin to run, be aware that your body may tell you it's not yet ready. For a few weeks after childbirth, as your uterus downsizes, your body will expel lochia, a brownish-tinged vaginal discharge, and this is normal. However, if it becomes too heavy or changes in color, alert your doctor. Bright red blood is a warning sign that you are doing too much too fast.

Don't rush to lose weight. A healthy diet and gradual return to exercise will allow the weight to come off when it is ready. Depriving yourself of calories or returning to exercise too soon to try to speed this process will only add stress to your new life. Keep in mind that all the changes your body went through for nine months can't simply be reversed in a month.

Postpartum Tips for Running

- Keep fluid intake high, and strive for pale yellow urine.
- Wear a very supportive bra, if not two, for the first several months particularly if you are breastfeeding.
- Start slowly and build. Don't expect to return to pre-pregnancy shape, speed, and mileage right away. Adding time to your run before speed will allow your body to adapt.
- Don't run so hard that you are too tired to be a mom. Use running as a positive energizer, not as an activity you have to recover from. Stop immediately if there is an increase in bleeding or if you have pain.

BREASTFEEDING AND RUNNING

It is completely safe and healthy to make running a part of your life while you're still breastfeeding. The most difficult issue for moms during breastfeeding is wedging in any activity at all between feedings. In the early months of a baby's life, you may feel overwhelmed with the demands of a nursing schedule and running may not be an option. Then, as time between feedings becomes greater, running provides an opportunity to use your body to nourish you. A recent Canadian study showed that running while breastfeeding can have positive effects on your infant's brain development. So if you can make the time, you will be reaping the benefits for both you and your baby.

Running Safely and Comfortably

It can be uncomfortable to run with full breasts, so if possible feed your baby before heading out the door. Make sure to wear a quality sports bra or even two to support your breasts. If your nipples are tender from breastfeeding, try applying a lanolin-based product to prevent chafing while running.

Keep in mind that breastfeeding requires an intake of an additional 300 calories per day. That means that if you are running, you will now need to take in additional calories to produce milk for your baby and also to keep yourself nourished. This is a critical time to make sure you are eating enough and not neglecting your own needs.

Also pay close attention to replacing whatever water you may have lost while exercising. If you notice that you aren't producing enough milk for your baby or if your urine is concentrated or dark, it may be a hydration issue, and you should try upping your water intake. An old trick is to drink a glass of water every time you feed your baby to keep from becoming dehydrated.

You may have heard stories about babies turning away from a mom's breast because post-run breast milk is soured by lactic acid. Though a small amount of lactic acid will exist if you've exercised at high intensity, your baby will not be aware of any taste difference, and there is no risk for either of you. If your baby seems to withdraw from the breast, it is more likely that it is the saltiness from your sweat, which can be fixed with a simple post-exercise wipe of your breast with a washcloth.

RUNNING AND MENOPAUSE

Menopause certainly has its advantages when it comes to running. There's no more worrying about your period on race day or stashing tampons on training runs. Menopause, which typically begins in the late forties or early fifties, is the last great cycle of a woman's life. It's a time that can make you feel really free, horribly sad, or any combination of emotion as the hormones that allowed us to carry children now begin to leave our bodies.

Women's experiences with menopause are as diverse as any other cycle of a woman's life. Some women will fly right through it and others will be affected by every symptom: hot flashes, irritability, anxiety, loss of sex drive, difficulty concentrating, hair loss, breast tenderness, and bloating. Pretty much any awfulness and awkwardness that a woman can experience is exacerbated in menopause. But running can help. There are no restrictions with menopausal running as there are with pregnancy or postpartum, which is a great start.

How Running Will Help Menopause Symptoms

- Weight control: As your body adjusts to this new stage of life, menopause can add unwanted weight. Combined with a strength-training program, running will help a woman retain muscle tone and a higher metabolism, which helps to keep weight in check.
- A brighter outlook: Running can clear a cloudy mind, turn away negative thoughts, and raise your spirits when the symptoms of menopause get you down.
- Better sleep: Menopausal women often have difficulty sleeping with or without night sweats. Maintaining a regular running routine will help aid in your

sleep, and if you are sleep deprived it will energize you during the day to bridge the gap until the evening.

- Heart health: The loss of estrogen during menopause negatively affects the good blood vessels. Running will help keep cholesterol in check when the estrogen levels drop off in menopause.

- Tougher bones: Unfortunately with the loss of estrogen, menopause increases the risk of osteoporosis. Running is a weight-bearing exercise so it increases the density of our bones and can be our way of fighting back. The National Osteoporosis Foundation recommends doing 30 minutes of weight-bearing exercise most days with at least two days of strength training per week to maintain good bone health, and the training program in this book will keep you on target.

SEE MOM RUN

Just less than a half century ago it was believed that running was detrimental to a woman's health. Fears of compromised fertility, sagging breasts, and collapsing uteruses have now been replaced with thoughts that running can prevent PMS, promote a healthy pregnancy, and assist in alleviating postpartum depression. We have come a long way in understanding the positive mental and physical benefits of running for women. As mothers, running provides so much more than a way to get in shape. It can be an outlet for stress relief, a re-energizer from a fragmented day, and a time to be alone or a respite with friends.

You are now armed with the why, when, where, and how of running, so now it's time to get busy and to *See Mom Run!*

REAL MOMS RUN

I run with a small group of gals. We're all moms with same-age kids. We're all at different levels, but find such support from a strong friendship built on endorphins and very funny group texts that leave us more sore from laughing than running. We've trained for and ran many races together.

—Jennifer, 34, two kids

PART 2

See Mom Train

"If what you are working for really matters,
you will give it all you've got."

—Nido Qubein, motivational speaker

CHAPTER 4

Training

The kids are asleep, at school, or in good hands; your shoes are tied, your mind is filled with the mental and physical benefits of heading out the door, and now what? You want to run, but now you need to know how much, how fast, and how far. Running will be a lifelong activity, as long as you respect your body and respond to its needs through cross-training, sound nutrition, and understanding when a niggle might be an injury. With this training program you will learn how to put a purpose to your run and how to prepare your body to move in a safe, progressive manner. The end result is getting you ready to run a 5K race, or 3.1 miles. (Though 5K sounds cooler, don't you think?)

The 5K is the most popular race distance in the United States, largely because it is a goal that is attainable without requiring many hours of training. It invites a new athlete to experience a race setting without overcommitting, and it allows more seasoned athletes to challenge their speed without taxing their bodies. But what if you don't want to run a 5K? That's totally acceptable, and the fundamentals of training still apply. You will still need to learn to respect your body as the vehicle. This is the body that you get. There's no trade-in or new lease.

There are four different training programs designed to progress you safely, and to make it child's play, I've named them after a baby's progression to walking: You must Creep before you Crawl, and you must Cruise before you Climb. After completing any of these programs, I hope you will be inspired to challenge yourself to toe the starting line and from there continue your running journey. Whether or not you are preparing for a 5K, you will learn the proper fundamentals for your stage of locomotion that best fits your current level of fitness. Creeping, Crawling, Cruising, or Climbing, there is a program that helps you achieve your goal. Please remember that before you get started in any exercise program it is important to consult your physician.

LEARNING TO TRAIN

Everything we do for our children, we do for a reason. We teach them to brush their teeth so they don't get cavities, look before they cross the street to be safe, or study for an exam with flash cards so they can pass a test. After some practice, our children begin brushing, looking, and studying on their own without question (at least the first two). It is similar with running. You need to learn it and practice before it becomes comfortable and routine.

Training for a 5K is doable in a mom's busy life. It doesn't require hours a day, yet it is enough to refresh, re-energize, and accomplish a goal without taking over your life. A 5K race doesn't take years to achieve; for most of you it will take three months or less. Once you cross the finish line, it isn't necessary to have more 5Ks stacked up on the calendar to keep running. Don't feel pressured to announce a yearly race circuit and spend your vacations running. Often one race is enough to introduce running to your weekly routine and give you the confidence that you can do it.

If you are apprehensive about competing in a 5K, you should begin with the training programs in this chapter, and learn to enjoy running. Then as your running progresses you may find the challenge of a race a nice reward to your training. Many 5K races offer week of or race-day registrations, so you might not have to decide immediately, though you might pay a premium by waiting. If you do decide to race, the training programs are helpful in keeping you on task, and attending the race puts you among excited, vibrant, and healthy individuals. A race will let you experience the thrill of adrenaline and self-accomplishment as you cross the finish line. The success will be all yours.

It takes about three weeks for your body to acclimate to a habit. The training programs here last six weeks at minimum, which is enough to cement a solid running routine and incorporate the time necessary into your daily life. If you complete your six weeks and run a 5K, and find that you enjoy running, you can remain in your selected program as long as you are comfortable or still feel challenged. If your running has progressed and you would like more of a challenge, then you can graduate your training to the next level. And conversely, if you don't want to race, use the program escalation to stimulate your running. This keeps you challenged in both mind and body.

Part of creating a running habit will be scheduling your workouts into your daily routine. It is just as important, however, to write down what you have accomplished. You can log your miles in a smartphone or use a traditional calendar. On those days that you struggle, look back at your calendar of workouts so you realize how far you have come in your training. Chronicling your workouts is also a helpful tool for workout compliance; you can record the time of day, weather, how you felt, what you wore, how far you went, and the time you walked or ran. This sort of running reflection helps to enforce the habit.

And remember, there are some days you might not be able to get the workout in—your child is needy, you have overwhelming work demands, you are under the weather, or all the above. Don't let that stress you out. It's okay to take an unscheduled day off or to complete a partial workout. You can always commit yourself to start fresh the next day.

Now, let's get moving!

GETTING STARTED

Take a moment to read through all the programs before choosing a correct starting point for you. The choice is not about where you want to be, not about where your friends are starting, but about being honest with yourself about your current fitness level. Be conservative at first, and you will be more successful. Training programs fail if you do too much too fast and can lead to burnout and injury. The programs are six weeks in length, geared to getting you to the starting line of a 5K race, confident that you will finish the distance within the guidelines of the training program you choose.

The training programs don't require a degree in astrophysics to learn to run. They are not designed to be supertechnical or overwhelming. The workouts are meant to fit neatly into one hour, several times a week, and will build confidence to completion. As the programs' levels increase, your speed will too. Measure your workouts in minutes not miles, as it is important to move your body for time, especially if you are new to running. The distance will come as you become efficient in the time allotted.

CREEPING PROGRAM CHECKLIST

The Creeping Program prepares you to walk a 5K in six weeks. It was impossible for your child to go from sedentary to crawling. Her body needed to prepare her muscles and bones to be strong enough to carry her weight on all fours. To begin a running program, you must prepare your body the same way. If your goal is to run a 5K, but you are new to exercise entirely, then please allow yourselves twelve weeks to your goal race.

Start with Creeping If:

O You have never run and/or have never exercised.
O You are just returning to exercise after a long sabbatical.
O You have a BMI (body mass index) of 30 or higher.
O You have difficulty talking or are breathless while walking in daily life activities.
O Your goal is to complete a 5K by walking briskly.

CRAWLING PROGRAM CHECKLIST

The Crawling Program prepares you to run a 5K with scheduled short walk breaks. As you progress through the Crawling Program, you will be able to determine a run/walk interval that works for you.

Start with Crawling If:

- ○ You used to run but have taken time off.
- ○ You currently have an aerobic base, but it isn't running.
- ○ You are interested in completing your first 5K utilizing a run/walk method.
- ○ You completed the Creeping Program successfully and are ready to progress to running.

CRUISING PROGRAM CHECKLIST

The Cruising Program prepares you to challenge your running effort and to run a 5K. This program introduces the Steady State Run (SSR)—a consistent run effort followed by a recovery jog.

Start with Cruising If:

- ○ You have recent running experience and want to run your first 5K race.
- ○ You have been running at the same pace and want to challenge yourself a bit.
- ○ You don't know how to organize your running and are looking to maximize your running time.
- ○ You have successfully completed the Crawling Program.

CLIMBING PROGRAM CHECKLIST

The Climbing Program prepares you to run at a personal best time in a 5K. This program utilizes strides, steady state, and interval running to strengthen your body and increase your speed and endurance.

Start with Climbing If:

O You have run for several years and are injury-free.

O You have 5K experience and want to run a personal best at the 5K distance.

O You have at least a year of consistent running, averaging 15 miles a week.

O You have successfully completed the Cruising Program and meet at least two of the criteria listed here.

REAL MOMS RUN

I mostly do run/walk intervals. I have run straight through workouts before, but I find that I enjoy the running much more when I break it up with consistent walk breaks. I also find that my average pace is a lot faster with intervals.

—Sandy, 32, one kid

THE PROGRAMS

The programs are broken into different days of the week with different tasks for each. There are days to walk and run, strength- and cross-train, and some that are designated for rest and recovery. On the left side of the table are the six weeks of training, and across the top are days of the week. Some people like to start their weeks on Sunday, others on Monday, so they are listed as Day #1, Day #2, and so on. If you need to rearrange the workouts to suit your schedule, that's fine, just try not to do two of the designated run days in a row, especially if your body is new to exercise, you are overweight, or if you need a little extra time recovering from exercise. You will find more information about the strength-training exercises in Chapter 5.

Your goal for the trainings should be to excel at running and to understand how your body reacts to running, so cross-training by doing another new exercise will make it hard to determine what might be bothering you if your body isn't responding well. You will want to know that when you are sore, it is directly related to something you did in this program. It's okay to be flexible. If you need to take a day off, then take a day off, but just make sure you're ready to get back out the door the next day. As you become more comfortable with your running, you can choose other exercises that challenge your body differently. For now, remember that you are a runner.

THE ESSENTIAL WARM-UP AND THE COOL-DOWN

No matter the program you choose, the warm-up and the cool-down of any workout remain the same. These are the bookends that keep your running injury-free, your joints firm, and your muscles supple. Your body needs this routine. If you are short on time, do not skimp on either piece, as both the warm-up and the cool-down are still active exercise. You will continue to burn calories, keep your heart rate elevated, and achieve the benefits of a workout.

Dynamic Warm-Up

The Dynamic Warm-Up prepares the body for running by using continuous movement to increase the blood flow to your arms and legs. The exercises are "dynamic" because you are moving your body, rather than remaining static, like traditional stretching. It used to be that we started every exercise with a lot of stretching, pulling, and tugging at cold muscles to prepare them for movement. It is better to bring your heart rate up gradually, which then delivers blood flow to your muscles to prepare them to run, and to avoid injury. Start all workouts with a walk or light jog before beginning the Dynamic Warm-Up.

The following exercises should take no more than a few minutes to perform and should be done after the prescribed warm-up in your program. Not every exercise needs to be done every time you exercise, but throwing in several of them will help prepare your muscles for your run:

- **100 Ups:** This is the simplest way to elevate your heart rate and to remind your body how to run. The 100 Up exercise is a slow-motion, overly exaggerated run in place. Standing tall, raise one knee to the height of your hip and back down, alternating legs. When one knee is up to hip height, briefly pause so that you are using balance to maintain your stance. Use your arms as if you were running. Repeat 100 times. As you get better you can pick up the speed and complete the exercise so that for a brief second neither foot is touching the ground. Make sure you are standing straight, with your core engaged and bringing your knee up to hip height.
- **Runner's Lunges:** Using an exaggerated first step, reach your left leg out, step forward, and lower your body down so that your left thigh is parallel to the floor. Your knee should be directly above or slightly behind your ankle, and your right leg should be stretched out behind you. Keep your core muscles tight so that you are keeping your back straight and tall. Bring your right arm up and left arm back as if you were running. Step up with the right leg and into the next lunge, moving your arms accordingly. Complete 10 lunges per leg.
- **Leg Swings:** Stand tall with your legs shoulder width apart and your hands at your waist or out to the side for balance. Lift one leg up to the side and swing it across the front of your body. If you have trouble balancing, perform swings holding on to a chair. Complete 10 swings on each side.
- **Butt Kicks and Knee Hugs:** Move forward exaggerating the back part of your walk by trying to kick your backside. Then bring your knee forward and up to your chest and hug your shin as you step forward. Complete 10 butt kicks and knee hugs for each leg.
- **Toy Soldier Walk:** Walk forward lifting one leg straight up to touch the opposing hand. Keep your ankles flexed and the lifted knee straight. Do not bend

your upper body or at the hips to reach your foot. If you can't touch your foot, just try to get as close as possible. Complete 10 per leg.

- **Hurdle Walk:** As you are walking forward circle your leg up, as though you are climbing over an imaginary log in the woods or a hurdle on a track. Walk forward and complete 10 hurdles per leg.
- **Calf Rolls:** Walk forward and roll your foot from heel to toe while you step. At the top of your step, rise up onto the ball of your foot and step forward with the other leg doing the same. Pump your arms as you walk. Walk forward and complete 10 rolls per leg.

Cool Down

Warming up gets your body started before you exercise, but it also needs to cool down when you're finished. If you finish your run at the front door of the house and plop down on the couch or jump directly into driving the carpool, you aren't allowing any of your systems to cool down. If you stop too quickly, you do not give your circulatory system the appropriate time to return to normal and this can leave you feeling faint or lightheaded.

Cooling down can be as simple as finishing your run with a light jog or brisk walk for 5 to 10 minutes. A more intense workout like the Cruising or Climbing Programs may require a 10-minute jog progressing to a walk for 5 minutes, while the Creeping and Crawling Programs may only need a few minutes. The goal is to return to regular breathing before ending the cool-down.

Stretching is a great addition to a cool-down and should be done after you have walked and returned your body to its pre-run state. While it is most important to cool down by walking, you may find you enjoy the stretches, so here are a few to try:

- **Knee Hugs:** Stand tall and walk forward lifting your flexed leg up and "hugging" it to your chest.
- **Behind Leg Grab:** Stand tall and walk forward, this time grabbing your leg from behind, with your hand grasping your ankle and keeping your knee pointed down.

- **Squat Leg Stretch:** Holding on to a chair or rail if you need balance, cross one leg over the top of your other knee and squat back as if you are sitting in a chair.
- **Inside Thigh Stretch:** Lunge to the side, keeping your knee over the top of your foot and the opposing leg straight.
- **Hip Flexor Stretch:** Step forward into a lunge with your hands on your hips or reaching straight up over your head and keeping your back leg straight. Raising and lowering your heel will also stretch your calves.

Your workouts should be viewed as three components: the warm-up, the run, and the cool-down. All are equally important to your fitness, improving balance, strength, and promoting an injury-free body. The more intense the workout, the more important it is to allow appropriate time to warm up and cool down.

CREEPING

The Creeping Program is about establishing the routine of exercise and preparing your body to run. You must first become adept at creating the time, stepping out the door, and then readying your body for the stress of running. For the six weeks of the Creeping Program you will be exercising up to six days, but with an emphasis on four workouts per week. Developing consistency is the key to a successful exercise program. While the other programs focus on running, in Creeping you should focus on walking with an intensity that is comfortable for you.

Most of us walk a bit every day, so it might seem silly to think something so simple can be healthful, help you lose weight, or prepare you to complete a 5K, but it does. The Creeping Program incorporates walking that is more vigorous exercise than strolling at the mall or meandering around the neighborhood. As your body adapts to the daily movement, your joints and muscles begin to acknowledge the new routine and build the structure necessary to move a little faster, while your mind understands and acclimates to the commitment. Walking uses the same muscles as running, and you will be training them to move forward at a faster pace. Walking at a pushed pace elevates your heart rate and breathing, and triggers your body to burn fat as its fuel source. As you progress, your conversation pace will increase as your cardiovascular and respiratory systems acclimate to the exercise.

The six-week program starts with 20 minutes of walking and builds to about 70 minutes. Most 5Ks will take you between 40 and 50 minutes, but the additional minutes of walking will ready your body for the force of running and build your aerobic endurance.

Walk Days

Fitness walking is done with purpose, with the intention of raising your heart rate, not as if you are browsing the Macy's windows in the mall. As you learned in Part 1, stand tall, engage your core, look ahead, and move comfortably. If you want to pick up the pace, concentrate on increasing the cadence (how quickly you step), not the stride length. Use your arms. Fitness-walking arms should be just the same as running arms, bent at 90 degrees and swinging front to back, not across your body and not down at your sides. By using your arms you will be utilizing your core and upper body, which will encourage you to stand tall. Use your toes, feet, calves, glutes, and core to move you forward, keeping a nice forward lean. The forward lean keeps you from landing flat on your feet, which slows your stride, and this position closely replicates how your foot lands while running.

On fitness walk workout days, you should move at a conversation pace, paying attention not to overwalk or become out of breath. Remember: If you can't answer questions in full sentences, you are moving faster than your body is ready to move. On the other hand, the easiest mistake is to walk at a rate that doesn't challenge you; if you find yourself disengaging from the task at hand, pick up the pace. Fitness walkers should strive for a 12- to 20-minute mile, depending on your starting level of fitness. To gauge how fast you are walking, try timing yourself at a track or a measured 1-mile distance. You should complete a fitness walk workout feeling like you exercised, not just like you came in from an evening stroll. Don't be afraid to work up a sweat.

Strength Days

As you begin to spend more time on the road you will get naturally stronger, and the addition of strength days will continue to aid in preparing your body to move. This simple strength program will take you less than 20 minutes in the first weeks, and as you progress to two or more sets of the workout it will take about 30 minutes. If you master these preparatory exercises and want more of a challenge, choose two other exercises from the Pick Six Strength Training Program in Chapter 5 to add to the workout.

Begin each strength day with a 5-minute walk. Walking for 5 minutes may seem silly and useless, but it is enough to remind your muscles of your new routine and warm them up for the strength routine. If you can't get out walking, then walk in place and add in a few flights of stairs if you can. If you are home with your kids, include them in your exercise. They will love counting the repetitions, and it won't hurt them to see you move and to move themselves.

In weeks one and two, perform each exercise one time through, then in weeks three and four try each workout two times through, and finally progress to three sets for weeks five and six.

- **100 Ups:** This is the simplest way to elevate your heart rate and to remind your body how to run. The 100 Up exercise is a slow-motion, overly exaggerated run in place. Standing tall, raise one knee to the height of your hip and back down, alternating legs. When one knee is up to hip height, briefly pause so that you are using balance to maintain your stance. Use your arms as if you were running. Repeat 100 times. As you get better you can pick up the speed and complete the exercise so that for a brief second neither foot is touching the ground. Make sure you are standing straight, with your core engaged and bringing your knee up to hip height.
- **Calf Raises:** Stand with your feet hip width apart with the balls of your feet supporting you, with your heels off a step or stair. Raise yourself with your feet, up to your tiptoes, and then drop your heels below the step. Begin with both legs at the same time and as you get stronger, try one at a time. You will feel this in your calves. Start with 15 double-leg raises and progress to 15 single-leg raises.

- **Reverse Toe Raises:** Now change positions on the step with your body facing down the step. Put your heel on the step with the rest of your foot suspended. Bring your toes up (flex) and then extend them down so that your toes are pointing to the ground. You will feel this on your shins. Start with 15 double-leg raises and progress to 15 single-leg raises.
- **Runner's Lunges:** Using an exaggerated first step, reach your left leg out, step forward, and lower your body down so that your left thigh is parallel to the floor. Your knee should be directly above or slightly behind your ankle, and your back leg should be stretched out behind you. Keep your core muscles tight so that you are keeping your back straight and tall. Bring your right arm up and left arm back as if you were running. Step up with your right leg and into the next lunge, moving your arms accordingly. Complete 10 lunges per leg.
- **Bridges:** Lie on the floor on your back with your knees bent and feet flat on the floor. Place your hands on the floor along your body. Push your hips up so that only your heels and shoulders are touching the ground. Hold for 10 seconds and lower back to the starting position. Complete one set of 15.
- **Pushup Progression:** Lie down facing the floor. Place your palms on the floor at chest level. Push into your palms, lifting your body with your knees bent on the floor and your feet lifted toward the ceiling. Keep your back flat and abdominals engaged. Push up until your arms are completely extended and then lower yourself back down to the starting position. Complete one set of 15.
- **Plank Progression:** Lie down facing the floor. With your hands palm down, push your body up so that only your forearm and toes are touching the ground. Squeeze your glutes and engage your core so that your body resembles a straight, stiff plank. Hold that position for 30 seconds, and build to 60.

Rest Days

Use these days to rest or reset if you are tired or sore. If you are feeling strong and want to exercise, by all means walk, but at a leisurely pace with the kids or the dog. Make sure you save yourself enough to approach the next week well rested.

CREEPING PROGRAM

	Day #1	Day #2	Day #3
Week #1	**25 min.** Walk	Strength Training	**25 min.** Walk
Week #2	**25 min.** Walk	Strength Training	**30 min.** Walk
Week #3	**30 min.** Walk	Strength Training	**35 min.** Walk
Week #4	**40 min.** 7x (Walk 4 min., Walk Fast 1 min.), then Cool Down (5 min.)	Strength Training	**40 min.** 7x (Walk 4 min., Walk Fast 1 min.), then Cool Down (5 min.)
Week #5	**40 min.** 7x (Walk 3 min., Walk Fast 2 min.), then Cool Down (5 min.)	Strength Training	**45 min.** 8x (Walk 4 min., Walk Fast 1 min.), then Cool Down (5 min.)
Week #6	**40 min.** 7x (Walk 2 min., Walk Fast 3 min.), then Cool Down (5 min.)	Strength Training	**30 min.** Walk

Day #4	Day #5	Day #6	Day #7
Strength Training	Rest	**30 min.** Walk	**20 min.** Walk
Strength Training	Rest	**35 min.** Walk	**25 min.** Walk
Strength Training	Rest	**40 min.** Walk	**30 min.** Walk
Strength Training	Rest	**35 min.** 5x (Walk 4 min., Walk Fast 2 min.), then Cool Down (5 min.)	**30 min.** Walk
Strength Training	Rest	**50 min.** Walk	**35 min.** Walk
Rest	**20 min.** Walk	**15 min.** Walk	Race Day!

Race-Day Strategy

On race day, alternate between 2 minutes of walking and 3 minutes of fast walking. Repeat this interval for the first 2 miles. If you feel stronger, walk fast for the remaining mile. Make sure that you plan your intervals so that you can finish strong.

Creeping to Crawling

If you were able to complete the six-week Creeping Program walk with a 12- to 18-minute mile pace and without any pain, then you are ready to begin Crawling. This run/walk program furthers your fitness and takes no more time than what you have already been putting in to the Creeping Program. If you struggled to complete the workouts, there is nothing wrong with continuing to walk a few more weeks before progressing to Crawling. Walking done at a brisk pace provides great fitness benefits, and as you begin to adapt to the exercise, your body will become stronger. Any time you are out on your feet moving your body, your systems take notice.

Congratulations: You have made the time to change your life; now let's continue the movement by introducing the run.

CRAWLING

The Crawling Program uses a run/walk interval progression in combination with a strength routine for six weeks to prepare you to run/walk a 5K race. Run/walk intervals are the safest way to increase time and mileage. It is also a widely accepted way to run a race—even experienced marathoners and professional runners run and walk. The walk part of the training allows your body to rest, reset, and increase your duration of exercise without the stress of only running.

Run/Walk Days

All run/walk days should be started with a 5-minute warm-up and finished with a 5-minute cool-down. Most of the workouts can be completed in an hour or less with the warm-up and cool-down included in that time.

The run/walk program gently introduces your body to running. By utilizing intervals you will spend more time exercising and gradually build your running endurance, linking walks and runs together. You will always have a walk break in the Crawling Program; it is expected that you take them. If you begin pure running too quickly, you could get injured. On the schedule, a run/walk day will look like this:

- Warm up for 5 minutes by walking briskly, then perform a few Dynamic Warm-Up exercises to get your joints and muscles ready to move.
- Intervals: 8x (1 min. run and 3 min. walk)—you will run for 1 minute and walk for 3 minutes, and then repeat 8 times.
- Cool down for 5 minutes by walking briskly.
- Strength days: Choose from the Pick Six workouts in Chapter 5.
- Cross-train: Depending on how you feel, this day can be used as a cross-training day or a rest day if you need it. Remember, cross-training doesn't have to be a formal workout; it can be a walk, hike, or a pickup tennis game.
- Day off: Rest, because your body will need it.

CRAWLING PROGRAM

	Day #1	Day #2	Day #3
Week #1	**40 min.** 8x (Run 1.5 min., Walk 3.5 min.)	Pick Six	**50 min.** 10x (Run 1.5 min., Walk 3.5 min.)
Week #2	**40 min.** 8x (Run 2 min., Walk 3 min.)	Pick Six	**50 min.** 10x (Run 2 min., Walk 3 min.)
Week #3	**50 min.** 10x (Run 2.5 min., Walk 2.5 min.)	Pick Six	**50 min.** 10x (Run 3 min., Walk 2 min.)
Week #4	**50 min.** 10x (Run 3.5 min., Walk 1.5 min.)	Pick Six	**40 min.** 8x (Run 4 min., Walk 1 min.)
Week #5	**50 min.** 10x (Run 4 min., Walk 1 min.)	Pick Six	**40 min.** 8x (Run 4.5 min., Walk 0.5 min.)
Week #6	**35 min.** 5x (Run 6 min., Walk 1 min.)	Rest	**24 min.** 3x (Run 7 min., Walk 1 min.)

Day #4	Day #5	Day #6	Day #7
Pick Six	Rest	**40 min.** 20x (Run 0.5 min., Walk 1 min.), then 2x (Run 2 min., Walk 3 min.)	Cross-Train/ Rest
Pick Six	Rest	**40 min.** 20x (Run 1 min., Walk 0.5 min.), then 2x (Run 2.5 min., Walk 2.5 min.)	Cross-Train/ Rest
Pick Six	Rest	**40 min.** 20x (Run 1 min., Walk 0.5 min.), then 2x (Run 3 min., Walk 2 min.)	Cross-Train/ Rest
Pick Six	Rest	**45 min.** 20x (Run 1 min., Walk 0.5 min.), then 3x (Run 4 min., Walk 1 min.)	Cross-Train/ Rest
Pick Six	Rest	**42 min.** 20x (Run 1 min., Walk 0.5 min.), then 2x (Run 5 min., Walk 1 min.)	Cross-Train/ Rest
Rest	**20 min.** 4x (Run 4 min., Walk 1 min.)	**15 min.** Brisk Walk	Race Day!

Race-Day Strategy

On race day, plan on running for 5 minutes and fast walking for 1.5 minutes. Repeat this interval for the first 2 miles. If you feel stronger, you can pick up the pace for the remaining mile, but plan your intervals well so you don't get overtired.

Crawling to Cruising

You may find that the Crawling Program works well for you and you are enjoying the walk intervals in your workout. There is nothing wrong with staying with the Crawling Program and improving on it by picking up the pace of the run or even the walk. The run/walk intervals provide an excellent workout and are an accepted form of running. If you feel ready to graduate, then by all means, step up to the Cruising Program.

CRUISING

In the Cruising Program, you will begin to run for longer periods, and if you choose, you can alternate your walk intervals with easy jogs. Combined with cross-training and strength days, you will continue to increase your running economy and efficiency. The Cruising Program introduces a new type of training called the Steady State Run.

The Steady State Run (SSR) is a larger block of running time without a walk break. If you have graduated from the Crawling Program, this run should be at conversation pace. If you have a stronger run base and are looking to improve, then the SSR can be done at a faster pace, which is also called a tempo run. This pace would be slightly above conversational at an effort that feels slightly pushed, but maintainable for the time prescribed. This is what Cruising is all about.

This program can be used over and over again and will continue to provide results as you become stronger.

Run Days

All run days should be started with a 5-minute warm-up and finished with a 5-minute cool-down. Most of the workouts can be completed in an hour or less with the warm-up and cool-down included in that time.

Run/Walk Days or Easy Run/Run Days

These days will look like this:

- Warm up for 5 minutes by walking briskly or with a light jog depending on your fitness level. The goal is to get your heart rate moving and ready for the workout ahead. Complete Dynamic Warm-Up exercises for a few minutes to loosen up and prepare your body to run.
- Intervals: 8x (4 min. run and 2 min. walk or easy jog)—you will run for 4 minutes and walk or jog more slowly for 2 minutes, repeated 8 times.
- Cool down for 5 minutes by walking briskly.
- Strength days: Choose from the Pick Six workouts in Chapter 5.
- Cross-train: Depending on how you feel, this day can be used as a cross-training day or a rest day if you need it. Remember, cross-training doesn't have to be a formal workout; it can be a walk, hike, or a pickup tennis game.
- Day off: Rest, because your body will need it.

CRUISING PROGRAM

	Day #1	Day #2	Day #3
Week #1	**48 min.** 8x (Run 4 min., Walk/Jog 2 min.)	Pick Six	**49 min.** 7x (Run 5 min., Walk/Jog 2 min.)
Week #2	**50 min.** 8x (Run 8 min., Walk/Jog 2 min.)	Pick Six	**50 min.** 5x (Run 8 min., Walk/Jog 2 min.)
Week #3	**48 min.** 4x (Run 10 min., Walk/Jog 2 min.)	Pick Six	**48 min.** 4x (Run 10 min., Walk/Jog 2 min.)
Week #4	**42 min.** 3x (Run 12 min., Walk/Jog 2 min.)	Pick Six	**48 min.** 3x (Run 14 min., Walk/Jog 2 min.)
Week #5	**44 min.** 2x (Run 20 min., Walk/Jog 2 min.)	Pick Six	**50 min.** EZ Jog 10 min., then SSR Run 30 min., then EZ Jog 10 min.
Week #6	**40 min.** EZ Jog 5 min., then SSR Run 30 min., then EZ Jog 5 min.	Rest	**30 min.** EZ Run

Day #4	Day #5	Day #6	Day #7
Rest	Pick Six	**40 min.** 2x (Run 5 min., Walk/Jog 2 min.), then 1x (SSR Run 10 min., Walk/Jog 2 min.), then 2x (Run 5 min., Walk/Jog 2 min.)	Cross-Train/ Rest
Rest	Pick Six	**47 min.** 2x (Run 8 min., Walk/Jog 2 min.), then 1x (SSR Run 15 min., Walk/Jog 2 min.), then 1x (Run 8 min., Walk/Jog 2 min.)	Cross-Train/ Rest
Rest	Pick Six	**50 min.** 2x (Run 5 min., Walk/Jog 2 min.), then 1x (SSR Run 20 min., Walk/Jog 2 min.), then 2x (Run 5 min., Walk/Jog 2 min.)	Cross-Train/ Rest
Rest	Pick Six	**52 min.** 2x (Run 5 min., Walk/Jog 1 min.), then 1x (SSR Run 24 min., Walk/Jog 2 min.), then 2x (Run 5 min., Walk/Jog 2 min.)	Cross-Train/ Rest
Rest	Pick Six	**50 min.** 2x (Run 2 min., Walk/Jog 2 min.), then 2x (SSR Run 15 min., Walk/Jog 2 min.), then 2x (Run 2 min., Walk/Jog 2 min.)	Cross-Train/ Rest
Rest	**30 min.** EZ Run 10 min., then SSR Run 10 min., then EZ Run 10 min.	**15 min.** Brisk Walk	Race Day!

Race-Day Strategy

On race day, plan to warm up briefly before the start by walking or with a light jog. Once the race starts, ease into a nice pace for the first 10 minutes at conversation pace; then pick up the pace to a SSR that is comfortable. If you feel stronger, try picking up the pace for the remaining mile.

Cruising to Climbing

The Cruising Program will challenge you as you begin to piece together more solid periods of running. During the six weeks of Cruising you will find your pace and also learn what it is like to push a little harder at times. Once you have mastered this program, you may find yourself ready to progress to Climbing.

CLIMBING

The Climbing Program is for an experienced runner who already has a solid base of running, has run a 5K, and is looking to achieve a personal best time. If you have landed here because you are interested in doing the most challenging program but are not an experienced runner, please start with one of the other programs. Without a solid run base, it is not advised to do this type of speed work. The Climbing Program uses Steady State Runs (SSRs), which are longer blocks of running without a walk break, and speed work to achieve a personal best in the 5K distance.

Run Days

All run days should start with a 10-minute warm-up and Dynamic Warm-Up exercises and finish with at least a 5-minute cool-down. Most of the workouts can be completed in an hour or less.

In the Climbing Program you will be challenging your running with different speeds and efforts. The program includes an optional fourth day of running per week. The SSR becomes an important part of your program as well as striders and interval runs (called Speed Pace in the workout table) that will be performed at about 15 seconds faster than your current 5K speed.

Here's what your week should consist of:

- Striders: A strider is a quick burst of speed that activates and recruits your running muscles and helps to develop leg turnover and speed. They reinforce your leg strength and speed, improve your stability and coordination, and will help your running economy. Striders should be done on a flat, soft surface such as a track or on grass. They also can be done on a straight stretch of smooth road or sidewalk. Begin with a shorter distance, about 50 yards, and then as you become stronger you can increase the strides up to 200 yards. The days in which striders are included have approximate times listed, as you can choose to vary the amount, length of stride, and time of recovery to fit your training needs.

  » Start a stride by running easy and working into speed with a short, quick turnover for the first quarter of your distance.
  » Lean slightly forward and run tall and relaxed. Use your best running form.
  » Build your speed by lengthening your stride slightly and keeping your turnover high, reaching top speed through the middle two quarters of your distance. Run as if you are floating. This is not a sprint but a controlled effort.
  » Begin decelerating for the last quarter of your distance before slowing completely.
  » When the stride is completed, walk or jog easy to the start to recover.
  » Start with four striders at a shorter distance and as your fitness improves, increase the length and repetitions. Striders can be done at different times during your workout, but only after a complete warm-up. Striders are also great to incorporate into a pre-race routine.
  » Cool down for 5 minutes by walking briskly.

- Strength days: Choose from the Pick Six workouts in Chapter 5.
- Cross-train: Depending on how you feel, this day can be used as a cross-training day or a rest day if you need it. Remember, cross-training doesn't have to be a formal workout; it can be a walk, hike, or a pickup tennis game.
- Day off: Rest, because your body will need it.

CLIMBING PROGRAM

	Day #1	Day #2	Day #3
Week #1	**40 min.** 4x (SSR Run 8 min., Jog/Walk 1 min.), then 4 Striders	Pick Six	**30 min.** 10x (Speed Pace 1.5 min., Jog/Walk 1.5 min.)
Week #2	**50 min.** 4x (SSR Run 10 min., Jog/Walk 1 min.), then 5 Striders	Pick Six	**40 min.** 8x (Speed Pace 2.5 min., Jog/Walk 2.5 min.)
Week #3	**50 min.** 3x (SSR Run 13 min., Jog/Walk 1 min.), then 6 Striders	Pick Six	**30 min.** 10x (Speed Pace 1.5 min., Jog/Walk 1.5 min.)
Week #4	**55 min.** 3x (SSR Run 15 min., Jog/Walk 1 min.), then 7 Striders	Pick Six	**40 min.** 8x (Speed Pace 2.5 min., Jog/Walk 2.5 min.)
Week #5	**55 min.** 4x (SSR Run 10 min., Jog/Walk 1 min.), then 8 Striders	Pick Six	**30 min.** 10x (Speed Pace 1.5 min., Jog/Walk 1.5 min.)
Week #6	**35 min.** EZ Run 20 min., then 5x (Speed Pace 1.5 min., Jog/Walk 1.5 min.)	Rest	**35 min.** EZ Run

Day #4	Day #5	Day #6	Day #7
Pick Six	Rest	**50 min.** Run	Cross-Train/Rest
Pick Six	Rest	**45 min.** Run	Cross-Train/Rest
Pick Six	Rest	**45 min.** Run	Cross-Train/Rest
Pick Six	Rest	**50 min.** Run	Cross-Train/Rest
Pick Six	Rest	**45 min.** Run	Cross-Train/Rest
55 min. EZ Run 15 min., then 6 Striders, then 5x (Speed Pace 3 min., Jog/Walk 3 min.)	Rest	**15 min.** Brisk Walk	Race Day!

Race-Day Strategy

On race day, plan to warm up for at least 5 to 10 minutes, then do three to four striders and a few Dynamic Warm-Up exercises. Stay warm before the race. Start the race at your comfortable SSR pace, and build through mile two. If you feel stronger, you can pick up the pace for the remaining mile.

REAL MOMS RUN

While I cannot say exactly that I run—jogging may be closer—I began on the treadmill during my ongoing weight-loss journey. Speed was not the goal. I completed the 5K within my goal of one hour. The scary part was starting. My body is not young and it was a long time since I exercised regularly.

—Nancy, 63, three kids

CHAPTER 5

The Pick Six Strength Training Program

Pure running is a whole-body experience, though it is the major muscle groups of the hips and legs that benefit the most: your quads, hamstrings, glutes, and calves. The straightforward movement will strengthen the large muscle groups, though the smaller stabilizing muscles can weaken, which can lead to instability and injury issues. Complementary cross-training days are included in the training programs and can be used for exercises such as yoga, Pilates, swimming, tennis, or other exercises that require lateral movement. These cross-training exercises will strengthen your running and promote a healthy body. The key is remembering that the cross-training effort is meant to support your running, not override it. You are training for a 5K, and your focus should be on the walk, run/walk, or running effort you have selected. These cross-training days are optional, though you should try to move your body in some way, even if it's just a brisk walk.

Your strength-training days are also included in your training schedule. The Pick Six Training Program will complement your running in ways you will surely begin to see as you move forward through the training. Adding the exercises to your schedule is about creating balance and structure for your body, not about big biceps or six-pack abs. In order to pay it forward and invest in your body, you need to have strength and balance, a platform for daily life and also for running.

STRENGTH TRAINING

Many women shy away from strength training for many reasons:

- Fear of looking like Arnold Schwarzenegger and appearing "pumped up."
- Fear of exercising around mirrors and looky-loos at a health club.
- Lack of knowledge about which exercises to do or how to work a machine.
- The time it takes to strength-train when aerobic exercise torches more calories per hour.

Strength training positively affects your running and your overall body composition, and boosts your metabolism. Strength training, even if it is using your own body weight as resistance, increases your lean body mass while decreasing your body fat. Strength training creates the lean, mean running machine that enables you to run strong and use your muscles to burn up calories effectively.

Advantages of Strength Training to Increase Muscle Mass

- Muscle burns more calories than fat even at rest. When you have more muscle mass, you burn calories even when reading the children a bedtime story.
- Muscle takes up less surface area than fat, so pound for pound you are trimmer.
- Strong running comes from a strong body. Strength training helps you power up hills with ease and increases your running endurance.
- Injuries occur less when you are stronger. Strengthening the muscles around the knees and hips can decrease joint pain and prevent overuse injuries.

The Pick Six Strength Training Program was developed to address those very concerns. The exercises will promote a healthy and strong running body. You will not get bulky or manly muscles, just stronger and better muscle tone. It is a variable strength-training program that allows flexibility in your routine while still giving a whole-body workout. If you have struggled with going to the gym, or even completing repetitive strength programs, then Pick Six allows the spice you will need to accomplish the workout. These exercises are easy to follow, can be performed in a half-hour or less, and can be done in the privacy of your own home. You can even get your kids to do them with you.

If you are following the Creeping Training Program, your strength-training exercises are included in Chapter 4. As you get stronger you may choose to add Pick Six to your regimen, but for now, the strength exercises included in the Creeping Program best prepare your body for movement.

REAL MOMS RUN

A lot of people wonder why I run, and it's hard to explain. When everything is right and it's a really good run, it just feels like I am doing something my body was designed to do.

—Cathy, 44, two kids

Getting Started

Running requires your whole body to move and Pick Six follows the same principle. The program focuses on developing stability and balance with an emphasis on your legs and core muscles, and should be done twice a week to maximize the benefits of the program. None of the exercises are so strenuous that you won't be able to run the next day. If you are limited in time, they can easily be done after a running workout on the same day. In the Climbing Program, you may find that you need more than a day's recovery from your speed workouts, so combining those days with the Pick Six works well.

The exercises are simple and require only one small investment: a stability ball. A stability ball is also called a Swiss ball, exercise ball, or yoga ball, and is a large, soft plastic inflatable ball that comes in sizes measured by diameter from 45 cm to 75 cm (about 18 in to 30 in) They range in price from about $8 to $30 and can be purchased at most sporting-goods stores, department stores, or online. Most balls will have a size chart that correlates to your height. If you are able to sit on an inflated ball before purchasing it, make sure you are sitting comfortably with your hips and knees at 90-degree angles with your feet flat on the floor, as if you are sitting erect in a chair. When fully inflated, the ball should not depress more than six inches when you sit on it. If you are new to stability and strength exercises, start with a ball that has less air pressure as it will be easier to balance. As your fitness improves, you can increase the amount of air in the stability ball, which will make the exercise more challenging. If you want an extra challenge, you can also invest in hand weights. You won't need weights greater than ten pounds, or you can accomplish the same thing with large cans of stewed tomatoes or beans that you might already have in your cupboard.

Pick Six Basic Knowledge

A few terms you will need to know for your exercises:

1. Rep: Short for repetition, it is one single movement within a given exercise, from the starting position to completing the movement and returning to the starting position again.
2. Set: A completion of one exercise, generally 10 to 15 reps with minimal or no pausing.
3. Circuit: A series of exercises, one after another.

PICK SIX

Begin each strength workout with a brief 5-minute warm-up of jumping jacks, running in place, a brisk walk, or even any of the exercises from your Dynamic Warm-Up. If this is the first time you have done any strength-training exercises, start by doing one set for 30 seconds and as you master the program, begin increasing the time to 60 seconds. If it is easier to count reps, start with 10 and progress to 15 per each set. As you begin to master the exercises you can add additional sets, working up to three sets per exercise.

On strength-training days, pick two exercises from each of the three categories listed, for a total of six. Strength training can get tedious and boring, so these allow you to mix it up. The program will stay fresh as long you pick two different exercises from each category every strength day. Find combinations that motivate you.

For each exercise, start with the Master This version, or the most basic example of each exercise. You should spend the first two weeks of the program on that version before moving to the more advanced options, Progressions. Each exercise requires balance and muscle control, so make sure you are comfortable with the movements before adding weight or a stability ball.

Once you have chosen your six exercises, they should be completed in one of two ways:

- Try one to three sets of each exercise, striving for 15 reps (that is 15 for each leg if it a single-leg movement, completing each exercise set consecutively before moving to another.

Or

- Complete the six exercises as a circuit (again, striving for 15 reps per set), repeating the circuit two to three times.

For either option, give your body 30 seconds to 1 minute rest between sets. You may rest 1 to 2 minutes before changing to a new exercise. If you would like to use the Strength Training Day as an added cardio workout, simply shorten the time between sets and intervals, not allowing your heart rate to fully recover. This is a wonderful way to increase the intensity and burn a few more calories.

Choose two exercises from each of the following groups of exercises (for a total of six):

Group A: Limbs and Movers

A-1: Walking Lunges
A-2: In-Place Reverse Lunges
A-3: Romanian Dead Lifts
A-4: Sidestepping Lunges
A-5: Mountain Climbers
A-6: Pushups

Group B: Front Core and Hip Stabilizers

B-1: Stability Ball Lying Trunk Rotation
B-2: Planks
B-3: Side Planks
B-4: Stability Ball Catch
B-5: Inchworm to Pushup
B-6: Russian Twists

Group C: Back Core and Hip Stabilizers

C-1: Bird Dog on Floor
C-2: Supermans
C-3: Stability Ball Leg Curls
C-4: Bridge to Marching Bridge
C-5: Golfer's Pickup
C-6: On Your Mark, Get Set, Runner's Pose

Pick Six Workout Example

5 minutes of warm-up

1. A-1: Walking Lunges
2. A-3: Romanian Dead Lifts
3. B-2: Planks
4. B-3: Side Planks
5. C-5: Golfer's Pickup
6. C-6: On Your Mark, Get Set, Runner's Pose

EXERCISE DESCRIPTIONS

Please read through the exercise descriptions carefully to develop proper form and reduce the risk of injury. Our bodies often auto-correct to an easier stance because our core muscles are not strong enough to stabilize the correct form. Or rather, we get lazy and compensate. Try doing the exercises in front of a mirror until you have mastered the proper form so you can see exactly how your body is moving.

GROUP A:
LIMBS AND PRIMARY MOVERS

A-1: Walking Lunges

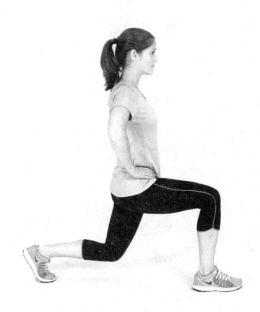

Master This:

- Stand with your feet hip width apart and your hands on your hips.
- Lunge forward with your right leg, bending your knee at 90 degrees. Your left knee should also be at a right angle behind you.
- Rise back up slowly, and step forward with your left leg to repeat.
- Continue forward, alternating legs with every step lunge.
- If you are limited in space, this exercise can be done standing and lunging in place.

Progression 1: Add Running Arms

- Perform the lunge as described, this time using "running arms."
- Use your opposite arms in running fashion to balance your legs.
- Flex your arms as you move them so that the movement is controlled and purposeful.

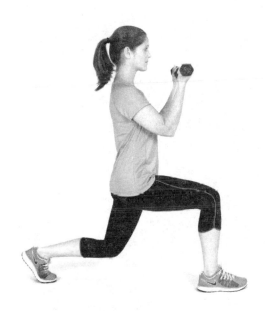

Progression 2: Add Dumbbells

- Begin with dumbbells at your side.
- As you step to lunge, bring your hands toward your shoulders, keeping your elbows next to your body.
- Return the dumbbells to your side as you return to standing and repeat.
- The exercise can be performed with both arms moving together or completing a curl with the opposing arm to the leg that is lunging.

A-2: In-Place Reverse Lunges

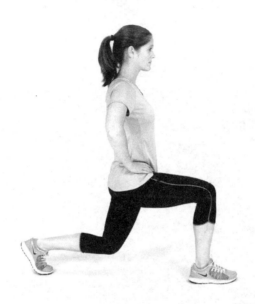

Master This:

- Stand tall with your feet hip width apart and your back straight.
- Step backward, dropping your back leg until your knee almost touches the floor.
- Your front knee should be directly over the foot forming a 90-degree angle.
- Return to the starting position by pushing off your back foot, using your glutes and hamstrings.
- Repeat the movement with your other leg, alternating each time.

Progression 1: Add Weights

- Hold weights in your hands while performing the previous exercise.

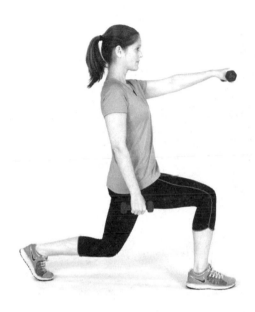

Progression 2: Shoulder Raise

- Begin with weights at your sides.
- As you lunge back, raise both your arms straight in front of you.
- Return your arms to your sides as you complete the lunge.

A-3: Romanian Dead Lifts

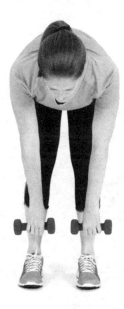

Progression 1:
Add Weights

- Perform the exercise with weights in both hands.

Master This:

- Begin with your feet shoulder width apart.
- Bend forward with your back straight. Hinge at the hip, pushing your bottom out behind you.
- Reach your hands down toward your toes.
- Squeeze your glutes and hamstrings, pushing your hips forward as you stand back up.

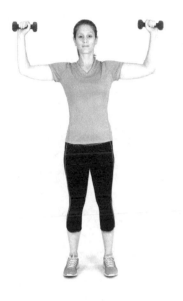

Progression 2: Shoulder Raise

- With weights in hand perform the exercise, but as you return to the start position, bend your elbows at the sides and raise the dumbbells to shoulder height with your palms facing out.
- Then press the dumbbells overhead, keeping your core engaged and shoulders down.

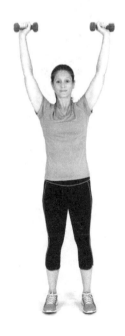

A-4: Sidestepping Lunges

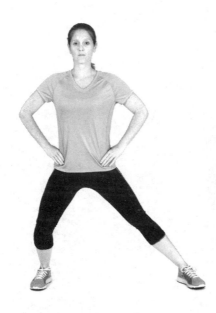

Master This:

- Start with your feet together, toes pointing forward.
- Step to the right, bending your right knee and shifting your weight to your right foot. Your left leg should be straight.
- Use your right leg to push back to the starting position.
- Repeat with your left leg.

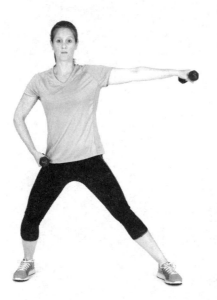

Progression 1: Lateral Shoulder Raises

- Hold a dumbbell in each hand at your sides in the starting position.
- As you lunge to the side, extend your arms, raising them to shoulder height.
- Lower your arms as you return to starting position.

A-5: Mountain Climbers

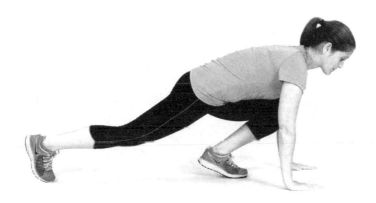

Master This:

- Start with your hands on the floor and arms extended in a top pushup position so that only your palms and toes are touching the ground.
- Hinge your hips so that your bottom is shaped like the peak of a mountain.
- Step one leg forward and the other back as if you are climbing up a ladder.
- Switch legs back and forth.

Progression 1: Increase Your Speed

- Pick up the pace so that you are "climbing" faster.

A-6 Pushups

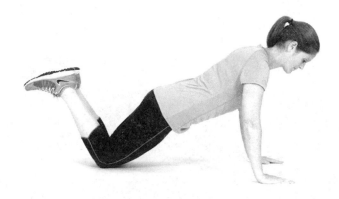

Master This:

- Start by facing the floor in a pushup position with your hands under your shoulders and your knees bent on the floor with your feet lifted toward the ceiling. Keep your back straight and squeeze your abdominal muscles.
- Lower your body to the floor by bending your elbows. Keep your body in a straight line.
- Return your body to the start position by pushing back up.

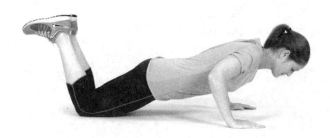

Progression 1: A Traditional Pushup

- Perform the same movement, this time with your legs out straight behind you and only your toes touching the floor.

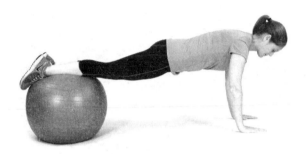

Progression 2: Add the Stability Ball

- Start in the upright pushup position, but balance your shins on a stability ball while performing the pushup.

GROUP B:
FRONT CORE AND HIP STABILIZERS

B-1: Stability Ball Lying Trunk Rotation

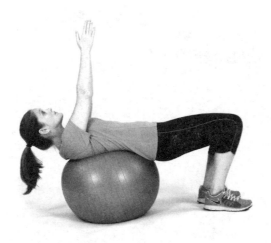

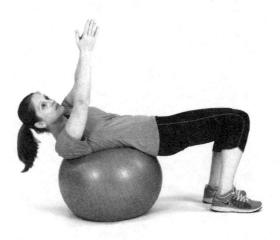

Master This:

- Lie down with your back on your stability ball and your knees bent at 90 degrees. Keep your hips up and in line with your body by squeezing your glutes and hamstrings.
- Extend your arms out above you, in line with your shoulders and keeping your elbows straight, and clap your hands together.
- Keeping your hands together, rotate your arms 45 degrees to one side while keeping your lower body still. Return your arms to the center and then rotate to the other side.

B-2: Planks

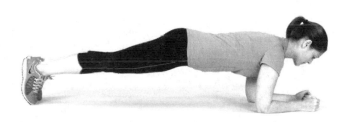

Master This:

- Start on all fours.
- Lower your body to your elbows so that they are directly under your shoulders with palms on the floor.
- Extend your legs out straight so that only your toes are on the floor. Your body should form a plank from your head to your feet.
- Squeeze your glutes and engage your core. Hold that position for 30 to 60 seconds.

Progression 1: Plank Toe Tap

- While in the original plank position, raise one foot off the floor and hold it for a few seconds.
- Perform the same movement with the other foot.

Progression 2: Plank Up Down

- Begin in the original plank position.
- Raise the right side of your body by putting your palm on the floor directly under your shoulder and straighten out your arm.
- Raise the left side of your shoulder in the same manner.
- Lower your body back down in the same sequence.
- Perform half the exercise beginning with the right arm, then switch.

B-3: Side Planks

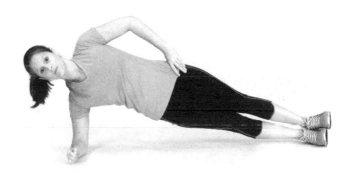

Master This:
- Lie down on your side and support your body on your elbow, directly under your shoulder.
- Position your arm that is on the ground so that your forearm is perpendicular to your body.
- Raise your body so that only your ankles and elbow are touching the ground.
- Use your free arm to stabilize your body if needed. Hold for 30 to 60 seconds.
- Switch sides and repeat.

Progression 1: Side Plank Up Downs
- Get into the original side plank position.
- Pulse your hips up and down slowly, keeping your core tight.

B-4: Stability Ball Catch

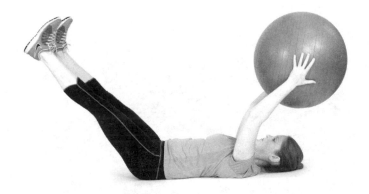

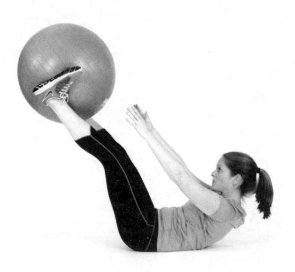

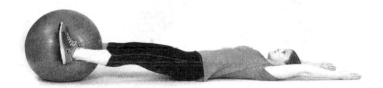

Master This:

- Lie down on your back, with your arms and legs extended with the stability ball in your hands over your head.
- Using your core, lift your straightened legs toward the ceiling while lifting your arms (and ball) up to meet them.
- Pass the ball to your feet, gripping the ball between your legs.
- Return your arms and legs to the floor, keeping them straight.
- Keeping your core engaged, return the ball to your arms in the same manner.

B-5: Inchworm to Pushup

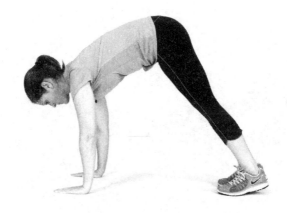

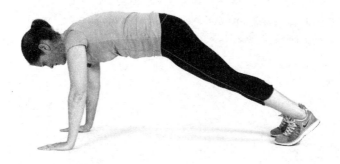

Master This:

- Standing tall, bend over and hinge at the hips.
- Reach to the ground. If your hamstrings are tight, bend at the knee so that your hands can touch the ground.
- "Inch," or walk, your hands out in front of you, taking small steps with your hands until they are in front of your head and shoulders. Use your core to keep yourself balanced.
- As soon as you are fully extended, take small steps with your feet back to the starting position.

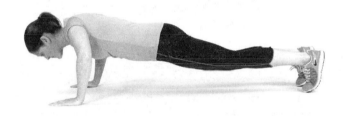

Progression 1: Pushup

- When you are in the flat-out position, lower your body to a pushup, then walk your legs back up to the starting position.

B-6: Russian Twists

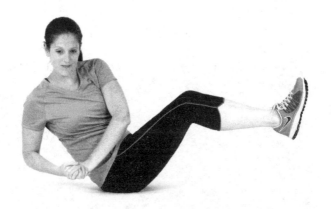

Master This:
- Sit down on the floor with your knees bent in front of you.
- Lean back slightly so your core is engaged and your back is straight with your elbows bent at your sides and your hands clasped together. Now, balance.
- Rotate your torso to the right, bringing your arms across your body, then rotate to the left. Return to the center to complete 1 rep.

Progression 1: Heel Lift
- Lift your heels off the floor slightly so that you are balanced entirely on your bottom, and complete the original exercise.

Progression 2: Add Weights
- Begin by holding one dumbbell between your two hands and as you get stronger add the second dumbbell. Hold dumbbells so that your hands or the weights are touching.

GROUP C:
BACK CORE AND HIP STABILIZERS

C-1: Bird Dog on Floor

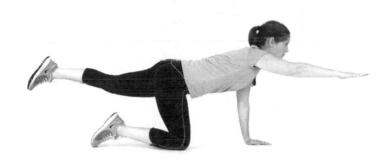

Master This:

- Position yourself on all fours on the floor.
- Simultaneously extend your right arm and your left leg (so that you look like a dog pointing to a bird).
- Using your core, balance yourself in the extended position for 5 seconds. Keep your hips stable and do not shift your weight to maintain posture.

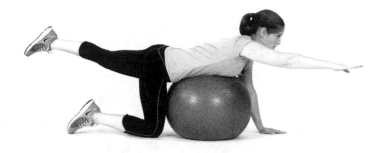

Progress 1: Add the Stability Ball

- Lay on the stability ball with the ball centered on your midsection. Place the stability ball underneath your core and perform the bird-dog exercise while balancing on the ball.

C-2: Supermans

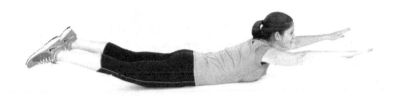

Master This:

- Lie face-down on the floor with your arms extended over your head and your legs out straight.
- Raise your upper torso and lower legs up off the floor so that you look like superman flying through the air.
- Hold yourself in this position for 5 seconds. Then return to the original position.

C-3: Stability Ball Leg Curl

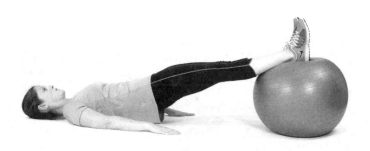

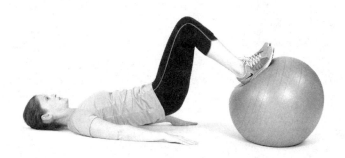

Master This:

- Lie on your back on the floor. With your knees bent, place your heels on the stability ball. Keep your hands at your sides on the floor to support you.
- Lift your hips up off the floor as you extend your legs out in front of you. Your body should be diagonally straight from shoulders to heels.
- Bring your heels back toward your bottom, then return to the starting position.

C-4: Bridge to Marching Bridge

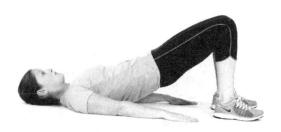

Master This:

- Lie on your back with your knees bent and your arms at your side.
- Lift your hips up toward the ceiling, making a diagonal straight line from your knees to your shoulders.
- Squeeze your backside and hold the position for 5 seconds before lowering yourself to the starting position.

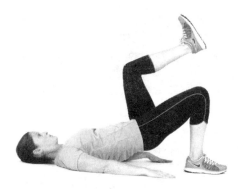

Progression 1: Marching Bridge

- Start in the original position.
- Lift one foot off the floor and hold your position without dipping your hips. Keep your core engaged.
- Repeat with your other leg.

C-5: Golfer's Pickup

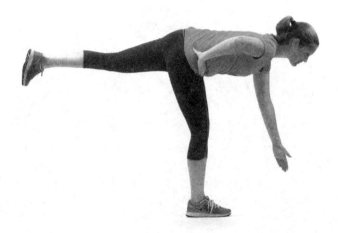

Master This:

- Stand with your feet hip width apart.
- Begin to bend at the hips and shift your weight to your right leg.
- Balance on your right leg, then tilt forward from your hips, lifting your left leg straight out behind you until your body is parallel to the floor. Create a straight line from your head to your foot.
- Reach for the floor with your left hand as if you are picking up a golf ball with your leg straight out behind you.
- Return to starting position, contracting your glutes as you lower your leg. Then step forward with your left leg and repeat the same movement. Alternate with each leg.

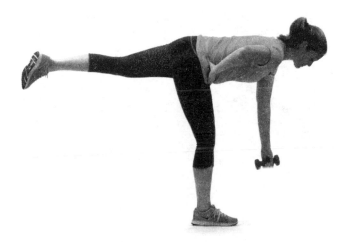

Progression 1: Add Weights

- Hold a dumbbell while following the steps in the original exercise. You can switch the dumbbell from hand to hand as you "pick up," or hold one in each hand, keeping the opposing hand at your waist with the dumbbell while extending the other hand and dumbbell.

C-6: On Your Mark, Get Set, Runner's Pose

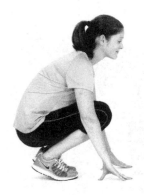

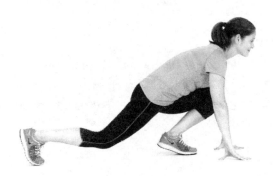

Master This:

- Step forward into a lunge position with your right leg, and lower your torso, placing both hands on the floor. Your left leg should be straight out behind you.
- Keep your bottom low and bring your left leg forward to meet your right, directly under your chest. Both heels should be on the floor.
- Extend your left leg back to the starting position and repeat for the remaining repetitions, and then switch sides.

MASTERING THE EXERCISES

You will have your favorite exercises in each category. These will come naturally to you, will be easy to complete, and will progress quickly. But it will be the exercises you struggle with that your body needs the most. Mastering the more difficult exercises—the ones you have a tough time completing or that make you feel wobbly and uncomfortable—strengthens the weakness in your body and also tests your mind. No one said this was going to be easy, but as you master and progress through these exercises, you will also see the improvement in your running, and ultimately in your goals.

REAL MOMS RUN

Running has benefited my life tremendously. It is free time, alone time, prayer time, and has opened my eyes to seeing the sunrise and sunset. It has helped me get through the mental stress of my company being sold and job elimination. It has helped me on my weight-loss journey by discovering that the scale sometimes doesn't move, but my pants and bra size can.

—Rachel, 43, two kids

CHAPTER 6

Eating to Train

No matter what you do, you can't outrun a bad diet. Late-night infomercials and bestselling books will tout the "secret" to the latest and greatest weight-loss tips, but they are mostly flashes in the pan. In truth, there is no secret eating methodology, no ancient potion, and certainly no pills that can ever supersede a simple, healthy lifestyle for you and your family. Every food you need to lead a healthier life, fuel your workout, and give you energy to get through a day, sleep better, and feel great about the body you have can be purchased at your local grocery store. Focus on fitness and health, and if you need to lose weight, it will happen as you begin to match your eating with your exercise.

PAYING ATTENTION TO YOUR DIET

We all can afford to eat a little better. As moms, we spend an inordinate amount of time making sure our children eat properly, harping on the virtues of veggies and the fineness of fruit, and yet our own diet consists of whatever we can eat while driving, folding the laundry, or muted on a conference call. Maybe it's the leftover waffles as you clear the table or the last bites of chicken tenders from a quick roadside diner, or if you are an eater like me, you nibble all day to ostensibly alleviate parenting stress. It's time to pay attention to yourself too. You mold your children with every bite you take and every bite that you don't. If you starve your own body to look better, you are showing them an unhealthy way to fuel. If you eat out of boredom or to relieve stress, you are showing your kids that food is not a fuel but a pacifier. It starts with you. As you begin this running journey, now is the time to make subtle changes that will be lasting eating habits to fuel you and your children for years to come.

Our diets really affect how our bodies respond to overall vitality, immune response, and disease. If you eat poorly, your body responds negatively. As you begin running you will be keenly aware of how food makes you feel. When you ask your body to perform it will start begging you to pay attention. If you think of yourself as a high-performance car, then regular fuel won't cut it. If you want to perform well, it is the high-octane fuel that will make that sexy engine purr.

Succeeding at eating healthy and fueling to run requires balancing input versus outtake. Think about your body as something that requires balance, like your money situation.

YOUR PAYCHECK

Let's say your family's paycheck comes twice a month, and let's assume the cash that goes into your account is enough to maintain your base living expenses—the mortgage, groceries, and your bills—to live comfortably. Without any major expenses catching you off guard, like your dishwasher breaking or needing a new muffler, your family gets fed, has a roof over its head, and your family life runs smoothly. Think of your paycheck as your base metabolic rate (BMR).

Your BMR represents the caloric intake you need to maintain all body systems at rest. So just like your paycheck, it is the amount you need to survive. The USDA's 2011 guidelines suggest that women aged twenty-six to fifty consume 1,800 calories per day (with a variance of 200 calories higher or lower depending on current muscle mass and level of activity). For this example, let's say that you need to eat 1,800 calories every day to maintain your current weight, similar to how your paycheck maintains you current lifestyle.

Now, as you begin to exercise, your body needs more energy to cover the calories you have used for the run. For example, to burn 300 calories, you might walk at a pace of 15 minutes per mile for 3 miles or run at a pace of 10 minutes per mile for 30 minutes. Now you must eat 2,100 calories to maintain your weight. If this was an extra expense in your life, you would have two choices: find a way to use your paycheck, or take out a loan that has a good interest rate. But what does that mean exactly for calories?

If you are interested in losing weight, then you should use your paycheck, and not replenish the deficit. In other words, this means that you should keep your calorie intake exactly the same. If you continue to take in 1,800 calories, your body will dip into your fat stores to cover the expended calories, and you will lose weight. If you want to maintain your current weight, then your choice would be to take out the loan. You will need to add calories to replace those lost in your workout. If you continue to eat the same amount as you did prior to exercise, your body will need 300 extra calories to maintain your BMR..

As you progress in your running program and your body acclimates to the exercise, you will be adding lean muscle mass, which increases your BMR. So, you actually get that cost-of-living increase by moving your body. Muscles drive your metabolic rate. More muscle mass means more calories needed, which means a higher BMR or an increase in your "paycheck." Everyone experiences a metabolic shift as we age, and some change with menopause, but we can slow the process by having an active lifestyle and maintaining muscle mass through running and strength training.

The Catch

The paycheck analogy only works to a point. Your mortgage, car payment, and credit cards don't care where the money comes from.

They just need to be paid, and money is money. But calories are not all necessarily the same. Even though your BMR needs about 1,800 calories, you will perform much better if those 1,800 are made up of fresh, nutritious foods, rather than doughnuts and soda. This will become much more apparent as you begin to run.

Your body demands better choices than junk food. In the short term, poor eating affects how you perform in daily life even without exercise. Poor food choices affect how you feel in the moment; how you respond to your kids; how you sleep; how your skin, nails, and hair look; and your overall well-being. Poor food choices today will affect your long-term health and longevity. To gain all the benefits that running has to offer, you must eat well. If you eat well, you will run well.

REAL MOMS RUN

I run so that I can eat whatever I want whenever I want. I run so that I am sane. I run because it is fun. I run because I've met the most amazing people through the sport. I run because it feeds my competitive side. I run because it is a part of who I am, how I see the world, and how I identify with the world.

—Nikki, 41, two kids

NUTRITION IN A NUTSHELL

According to the U.S. government, there are five food groups that we need to maintain a healthy diet. Not much has changed since elementary school except that a few of the food groups have been altered to encompass a healthier choice of food sources. The healthy diet contributors are: Fruits, Vegetable, Grains, Protein Foods, and Dairy. Including the five food groups in your daily diet is important, but you also need to keep an eye on the portions on your plate to ensure you are eating to promote a healthy body. The USDA recommends that our daily plate include fruits, vegetables, protein, grains, and dairy with a little bit of essential oils, based on your 1,800-calorie diet.

Tips for Filling Your Plate

- Make half your plate fruits and vegetables.
- Make half your grains whole grains.
- Choose lean meats, eat fish at least twice a week, and incorporate nuts and legumes as a protein source.
- Switch to low-fat dairy, but watch added sugar when selecting flavored dairy drinks or yogurt.
- Avoid saturated fats, trans fats, and cholesterol.

Check in on Your Calcium and Vitamin D

To keep up you bone strength and prevent osteoporosis, especially as you get older, it is very important to get all your calcium and vitamin D. The Institute of Medicine of the National Academies recommends a daily allowance of between 1,000 and 1,300 mg of calcium and 600 IU of vitamin D a day for women ages nineteen to seventy. As a frame of reference, a glass of milk contains about 300 mg of calcium and 100 IU of vitamin D. Calcium and vitamin sources, like fortified orange juice and cereals, can help bridge the gap of naturally occurring nutrients that can be found in dairy products, dark leafy greens, and fish.

POWER FOODS FOR RUNNING

The best way to eat a healthy diet and fuel your body for exercise is to shop the perimeter of the grocery store. The center aisles of a grocery store are filled with packaged and processed food, which are high in sugar and unnecessary ingredients to sustain a healthy life. The perimeter is where you'll usually find the produce, meats, fish, dairy, and the fresh bakery. It takes effort at first to train your cart not to dip into the chip aisle, but soon enough your body won't crave the empty calories.

To help you with your food choices and to gain a better understanding of which healthy foods to incorporate in your running life, Sotiria Tzakas-Everett, a sports nutritionist for the Women's Sports Medicine Center at the Hospital for Special Surgery, has offered ten power foods for running. All these foods are easy to find at most grocery stores and offer a great start to better nutrition and health:

1. **Fat-free Greek yogurt:** Thick, creamy, and filling with almost double the protein of regular yogurt, this delicious food is also a good source of calcium (about 200 mg) and probiotics, to keep bones and the digestive system healthy. Greek yogurt is also versatile. It can be used in fruit and vegetable dip recipes, as a sour cream alternative, or as a snack with some granola.

2. **Nuts and nut butters:** An energy-boosting, meat-free alternative for protein, while offering heart-healthy nutrients such as vitamin E, folate, and omega-3s, nuts are wonderful portable snacks, and nut butters can be included in sandwiches and baking recipes, added to smoothies, or mixed into oatmeal. Be mindful of portions, and choose unsalted raw nuts and nut butters without added salt and sugar.

3. **Dark leafy greens:** Leafy greens such as kale, spinach, and Swiss chard are often considered some of the healthiest foods since they are packed with a variety of vitamins (A and K), minerals (iron and calcium), fiber, and antioxidants. These greens are easy to prepare and can be eaten raw in salads, chopped and sautéed in olive oil, or even incorporated in fruit and vegetable smoothies.

4. **Beans:** Another versatile and meat-free protein source, beans, such as garbanzo, kidney, and black beans, offer the most fiber per serving of most other foods, to help keep you full and your gut healthy. They are also a source of important nutrients for active women, such as folate, iron, and magnesium.

5. **Blueberries:** This vibrant fruit is rich in polyphenols, which have anti-inflammatory and antioxidant properties, in addition to fiber and vitamin C.

Choose fresh when in season or frozen. Enjoy on their own, or as a topping for cereals and yogurt.

6. **Bananas:** A go-to food for many runners since they are high in carbs and potassium, and are easier to digest than some other fruit, bananas come in nature's perfect package and can be tossed into any bag, ready to eat before a run.

7. **Oatmeal:** Plain, old-fashioned oats are best to gain the fullest amount of fiber without the added flavors or sugar. Oatmeal provides long-lasting energy in the form of complex carbs and fiber, which is perfect before a workout. Cook with milk or a milk alternative to add calcium and protein.

8. **Flaxseeds:** Flaxseeds are an excellent source of omega-3s, plus fiber, protein, and potassium. Flaxseeds can be purchased whole or ground and make easy additions to baked goods, yogurt, cereals, salads, and smoothies.

9. **Fatty fish:** Fatty fish such as salmon, tuna, sardines, and mackerel are some of the best sources of heart-healthy omega-3s and healthy proteins. Buy them fresh or canned for an easy addition to salads and sandwiches. Canned sardines and salmon are also a source of calcium.

10. **Sweet potatoes:** Another low-fat, high-fiber healthy carb, sweet potatoes are rich in potassium and are a source of vitamin C and iron. Sweet potatoes can be enjoyed simply baked or roasted.

MACRONUTRIENTS

Every piece of food that makes up your plate is comprised of three different macronutrients: fat, carbohydrates, and protein. These macronutrients are all necessary components of maintaining a healthy diet, and all three are necessary to building a healthy running body. Relying too heavily on one food group or one macronutrient will not make you leaner, promote your fitness, or encourage great health benefits. To take advantage of the positive properties of food, you need moderation, balance, and a diverse diet. Deprive yourself of one nutrient and you will overcompensate in another, causing an imbalance. If you stop eating carbs, you won't think straight; give up protein and your body can't repair itself; eliminate fats and you lose vital body functions. Eat too many of them all and you gain weight. Excess calories make you fat. Eating the correct amount for your energy expenditure makes you fit.

If you are pregnant or breastfeeding, your body needs additional calories for the fetus or milk production, and those should be added to the calories allotted in your BMR.

Fat

Fat fights inflammation, helps with absorption of key vitamins, and balances hormone production, though it is often maligned because it shares the name with what most of us don't like to have on our bodies. Fat contains about nine calories per gram, while carbohydrates and proteins contain four, which is five calories too many when loading up on "fat-heavy" foods.

There are good fats and bad fats, but both should be eaten in moderation. The CDC recommends that fats make up 20 to 35 percent of your daily diet. The good fats—polyunsaturated and monounsaturated—come from nuts, fish, and vegetable oils. The bad fats—saturated fats, trans fats, and cholesterol—are often used by food manufacturers because they give food a longer shelf life. If they last longer on the shelf, imagine how long they last on your body. Remember: Fats do not make you fat, excess calories do.

Carbohydrates

Carbohydrates provide a short-term fuel source that provides energy to your cells and supports an active lifestyle. They also can be stored for later use and are typically the energy source your body calls on first when it needs fuel. Carbs are brain food, and without them you feel fuzzy and have difficulty making decisions. There are two types of carbohydrates: simple and complex.

Simple carbohydrates provide our bodies with sugar that is already in its simplest form so your body does not have to spend too much time converting them into fuel. Simple carbs offer a quick boost of energy, but they are also responsible for the quick low that follows, causing you to feel lethargic as your body tries to respond to balance the sudden spike of sugar. Examples of simple carbohydrates are processed foods like white breads, pastas, box cereals, cookies, ice cream, and regular soda. All these examples contain added sugars that increase your calories without any nutritional value. It would be easy to say that ridding your diet of simple carbs would be the healthiest option; however, there are essential simple carbohydrate foods like fruits, vegetables, and dairy products that provide our bodies with critical vitamins and minerals. It is best to keep the simple carbohydrates to those natural sugars and avoid the ones that come in manufactured or processed foods.

Complex carbohydrates provide your body with a fuel source that is broken down slowly, so they serve as a longer-acting fuel source. Examples of complex carbs are whole grains, legumes (beans), fruits, and vegetables, and all contain nutritional starches and dietary fiber that provide quality nutrition.

Many carb-free fad diets promote dramatic weight loss, something that happens as your body goes into a crisis mode, resorting to cashing in on fat stores but also utilizing muscle. The result is fast weight loss that is not sustainable. The American diet is full of simple carbohydrates—too much refined sugar, white flours, pastas, sodas, and snack foods. These foods provide fast energy and do little else to support your system and leave you hungry sooner. Search out complex carbohydrates that your body will work harder to digest, and you will feel satisfied longer. And remember: Carbohydrates do not make you fat, excess calories do.

Proteins

Protein is the builder and the healer for the body. It is the macronutrient that is the basis of our cell structure, not just in your muscles, but for your entire body. Protein helps repair muscles after they work hard and provides the foundation for building new muscle. Most commonly we think of meat as the greatest source of protein, but beans, nuts, eggs, dairy products, and seeds can also offer protein-rich alternatives. It is important to consider what comes along with the protein you choose. For example, if you only choose protein sources from a T-bone steak, then you will be consuming a lot of saturated fat, whereas a cup of beans provides protein, fiber, and minerals. Protein is found in cottage cheese, Greek yogurt, and even in a banana. Your body has to work harder to digest protein, so you won't feel as hungry after eating a meal with this macronutrient. Remember: Proteins do not make you fat, excess calories do.

WEIGHT LOSS

If you are interested in losing weight, an important step is to journal what you eat. A 2008 study by Kaiser Permanente's Center for Health Research found that people who maintained a food journal lost twice as much weight as those who didn't. What makes this so effective is accountability. You really start to focus on what you're putting in your body when you have to write it down.

There are hundreds of apps available or online programs that make tracking your food intake easy and motivating—for example, MyNetDiary. Like many others, this app can be used on a variety of computer and smartphone platforms and allows you to really see what you are eating and how exercise can play a role. These smart programs provide you with the nutritional breakdown of virtually any food and when used as a daily diary can show where the potholes exist in your diet. The program will tally your calories and also let you input your exercise. This gives you a complete look at how effective and important exercise is for weight loss. Many of the apps also have online communities that support your effort as you lose weight.

If you don't have access to a computer or smartphone, try journaling your daily food consumption in a notebook. Recruit a friend or family member to journal with you. Writing down what you eat makes you aware and responsible. Although it isn't always convenient, try writing down what you are going to eat before you eat it. For example, serve your plate and then make a quick note of your meal and commit to what is on the plate, and no more.

The training programs in this book will help you burn calories, stimulate your metabolism by building muscle, and give you the motivation to lose weight by introducing you to a healthier life. As you begin to make running a part of your life, your food choices will become wiser, and you will become aware of the influence that eating well has on your running. Match a healthy diet with a running program and you are on your way to more energy, more confidence, and being a healthier mom.

FUELING YOUR RUNS

Graduating from a sedentary woman with a caloric intake around 1,800 calories a day to a fabulous, fit, running mom requires more than lacing up sneakers. Though the number may differ slightly based on your size and build, a good rule of thumb is that you typically burn about 100 calories per mile. If you have an idea of how many calories you are burning each time you run, you can adjust your diet accordingly.

Aside from a balanced diet, the most important consideration in eating as an athlete is when to eat. Eat too close to exercise and intestinal distress cramps will ruin your run. Don't eat close enough to running, and your legs will run out of energy. Jennifer Hutchison is a sports dietitian who coaches elite athletes. If you find yourself struggling to understand when to eat or how soon after eating a meal you can run, she has shared few suggestions:

- **4+ hours before a run:** Eat a regular balanced meal—breakfast, lunch, or dinner consisting of 500 to 600 calories. The meal should contain a small portion of protein, such as cottage cheese, yogurt, eggs, or chicken, plus a serving of a wholesome carbohydrate source, like an English muffin, whole-grain bread, large potato, or a cup of rice or pasta.
- **2–3 hours before a run:** If you are eating two to three hours before exercising, strive for a 300- to 400-calorie meal. A meal that has lean protein and quality carbohydrates will give you the energy to get out the door and running: Greek yogurt topped with granola, multigrain toast with peanut butter, or a balanced energy bar if you need a convenience food. Avoid foods that make you gassy, such as beans or dairy.
- **1–2 hours before a run:** Focus now should be on a carb-rich snack that is 100 to 200 calories, or basically what fits into the palm of your hand. Keep it carb focused, with a bit of protein. A banana with a smear of peanut butter, a handful of pretzels, or half an energy bar are all good options.
- **30 minutes before a run:** This is a good time to get in a quick snack that's fewer than 100 calories. Snack foods like individually packaged applesauce or a handful of nuts will be enough to fuel your run.
- **Minutes before a run:** Eating too close to running can be difficult on your digestive system, resulting in cramping, but not eating can be worse. If you find an opportunity to run but you haven't eaten, try getting 50 calories of quick energy. Eight ounces of a sports drink, a quick bite of the chocolate Easter bunny you found hidden in your kid's closet, or about thirty raisins will work. Or if you are an early morning runner and haven't eaten since the night before, four ounces of orange juice or a few bites of a banana will suffice.

WATER

Your body needs water for all bodily functions. Food is metabolized more efficiently when we are hydrated. Surprisingly, most of us are appropriately hydrated if we drink with our meals, maintain a diet rich in fruits and vegetables, and respond to our thirst by drinking water. If you keep a water bottle with you in the car, while you work, at the soccer field, or at home, it will remind you to stay hydrated. Choosing water, as opposed to other calorie-rich liquids like soda or sugar-added fruit juice, will aid in keeping your body properly hydrated and reduce empty calories.

Pay attention to your thirst throughout the day. Hydration shouldn't be left to the last minute—otherwise it will be sloshing around your gut as you run. You can drink up to eight ounces about a half-hour before running. If the weather is mild, it isn't necessary to bring water along if your run is less than an hour. When the weather is hot, carrying a bottle of water, stashing some along your route before you run, or investing in a hydration belt will keep you from becoming dehydrated. Responding to your thirst is the best way to remain hydrated.

But what about sports drinks? Major beverage companies put a lot of money into advertising their sports drinks, showing beautiful bodies guzzling these fluorescent liquids, leading us to believe that they are necessary for athletic performance. For the amount of running you'll be doing to train for a 5K, a sports drink is likely not necessary. They are made up primarily of fast-acting sugars and sodium to replace necessary electrolytes that are lost in perspiration. If you are running or completing endurance events lasting more than an hour, then a sports drink can help keep you hydrated and healthy, but for the *See Mom Run* training, it's probably better to skip.

Likewise, reserve sports bars for gearing up for a run lasting more than 90 minutes. You may come across energy gels, bars, and candies at running stores or your local grocery store. These items are geared toward a runner that is training for events over an hour in length such as a half marathon or triathlon. You won't need any of these things to train at this point of your journey, but sports bars are always good for a quick bite if you need them. Make sure to read the labels though, and be confident about what you're putting into your body.

RECOVERY FOODS

After a run, there is about a 30-minute window when your metabolism continues to burn calories at a higher rate. According to Sotiria Tzakas-Everett, sports dietitian at the Women's Sports Medicine Center at the Hospital for Special Surgery, this is also the time that your body will take fuel and send it to the muscles so they can recover for the next workout and the rest of your day. This does not mean you should fill up with empty or excess calories, but instead use that window to eat a quality source of protein and carbohydrates totaling 150 calories. Eating within a half-hour will also satisfy your hunger and give you a boost until your next meal. A favorite is eight ounces of low-fat chocolate milk, which tastes rich and rewarding. Other suggestions are cottage cheese or yogurt and fruit or an apple and a half handful of nuts. There's no magical nutrition solution, so be creative in your choices and make your 1,800-calorie paycheck count. Eat well, live well, run well!

REAL MOMS RUN

I think that there is not one single particular person who inspired me to run. Growing up, to be honest, I was bad at sports. With running, I can be by myself and I don't have to worry about hitting balls, catching balls, etc. I found that while running I can be athletic all by myself. I suffered from bad self-esteem growing up and running makes me feel so good. It gives me power and strength. It makes me feel like I can do anything!

—Kirsten, 38, two kids

CHAPTER 7

Injury Prevention

Running is stressful on the body. There it is, finally out in the open. The truth is that running is a delicate love, and you must respect it or lose it. Running injuries are not typically traumatic injuries, the type in which you break a bone or require stitches. More often they are overuse injuries, the result of running too many miles too quickly, running too fast, or running too often. The American Academy of Physical Medicine and Rehabilitation reports that nearly 70 percent of runners will become injured in their lifetime. If you balance your runs with the Pick Six Strength Training, cross-training, and rest days, you will develop into a more complete runner and greatly reduce the risk of injury.

Niggle

noun

: a slight feeling of something (such as doubt)

: a slight pain

: a small criticism or complaint

INJURY PREVENTION, OR KEEPING THE NIGGLES FROM GROWING UP

A niggle is the initial onset of a "too much" injury. A niggle doesn't wake you up at night or stop you dead in your tracks, but you can still feel it, and it's important not to let it go unattended. Almost every running injury begins as a niggle, something that may bother you a bit as you warm up and then subsides as you get warm. A niggle usually doesn't warrant time off, but it is a good idea to pay attention and evaluate the change that has happened in your running to cause the disturbance. If a niggle doesn't subside as you get warm, but rather increases in intensity, is persistent, or causes you to alter your gait, you need to stop and listen to your body. This is no longer a niggle; it is an injury. Here are a few rules for keeping things in check.

Warm Up

Beginning a run without bringing your muscles slowly up to speed will promote injury. Gently raising your heart rate, completing Dynamic Warm-Up drills, and increasing your pace slowly will allow your body to respond and decreases potential traumatic muscle pulls and stress on your tendons.

Know Your Roads

Your regular route can change in an instant if the seasons change, causing unsafe conditions. If it is icy, snowy, or slick out, even running with caution can be dangerous. This cautiousness can alter your gait and posture, which can lead to an injury. If you are running in an unfamiliar area, ask locals about the conditions of the roads so that you have an understanding if uneven, sloping road shoulders, traffic, or other obstacles may put you at risk of injury. If you are a new runner, sticking to flat, smooth surfaces is the best bet while your feet and ankle muscles build strength.

Understand Your Limits

If you chose a training plan that is too much and you are having a hard time recovering, your body is overly sore, you have residual pain the day after, or you are just exhausted, then an adjustment needs to be made. Not all plans work for all people. If Susie, your neighbor, convinces you to do the Crawling Program because she is using it and would love to have you as a partner, only commit if it is within your limits. As your training improves, you will be able to run longer and faster, but ease into it and injuries will stay away.

Keep to the 10 Percent Rule

When starting to run for the first time, don't increase your mileage more than 10 percent per week. Your body needs time to acclimate to mileage and does it best little by little. Running is a weight-bearing exercise, and your body absorbs two to three times its own body weight with each footfall. If you build your running too fast, your bones cannot compensate, and stress fractures can happen as a result. By increasing the mileage slowly, you will give your muscles, tendons, and bones a chance to build a solid running structure.

Don't Borrow Someone Else's Gait

Borrow maternity clothes, evening gowns, or a cup of milk from your neighbors, but don't borrow anyone else's gait. We all want to have the graceful form of an Olympian, but that style of running took years to perfect and is unique to the individual. You should run the way your body was meant to run, which means keeping to a stride that is comfortable for you. When your fitness improves, through consistent running and strength training, you can make subtle changes to your form. But keep your style your own and don't get distracted by trying to imitate other runners.

Vary Your Workouts

Too much of a good thing can lead to an injury. By including strength training and cross-training in your running routine, you will develop into a better runner. You will feel stronger, more rested, and ready to run.

Invest in the Right Gear

Do not run in cross-training shoes or your Victoria's Secret décolletage bra. Run in running shoes. Wear a supportive running bra. Find gear that is designed for running that is made to withstand the sport and will keep you cushioned and supported. Shoes generally last 300 to 500 miles, but always listen to your joints. They will tell you when to replace your shoes.

Make Nice with RICE

RICE is a simple way to prevent niggles from becoming injuries. It is an acronym that stands for Rest, Ice, Compression, and Elevation. Running niggles, especially overuse injuries, respond well to RICE, so it should be your go-to remedy. If RICE doesn't help after two to three weeks of diligent practice, then it is time to consult a sports-trained physician or physical therapist to get an evaluation. RICE is also a great way to treat injuries such as sprained ankles and really any bump or bruise that happens to you or your children.

- **Rest:** This could mean taking a few days off to rest the niggle, but keeping active as long as you're not in pain is fine. Cross-train, or try a slower or simpler route until you feel better.
- **Ice:** Applied several times a day, ice is an easy way to silence a niggle, and there are several ways to apply it properly. Fill a resealable bag with ice and wrap it around the injury with an elastic bandage or even a sock. Or if you need something cold in a pinch, use a bag of frozen peas or corn. Both

methods conform to your anatomy and can be continually reused. With either method, be sure not to apply the ice directly to the skin. Use a pillowcase or T-shirt to wrap the ice so that there is a barrier. Never leave ice on for more than 20 minutes.

Another option is to fill small paper cups with water and freeze them. Once frozen, tear the top portion of the cup down to expose the ice while still maintaining the base of the cup to hold. Use the ice cup to massage the niggle in a circular motion for 15 minutes. This "ice massage" will cause the skin to get red and feel very cold at first, but with the friction of the massage it will become tolerable.

- **Compression:** You may have seen people wearing technical clothing like knee-length socks or bike shorts. No, the eighties are not back. This compression gear can help support muscles during exercise and is also useful for injury recovery. Compression reduces muscle fatigue and supports your muscles during exercise. It's not necessary to buy expensive compression gear, since you can achieve the same results by applying an elastic bandage to help a niggle feel loved. If you are wrapping a body part in an elastic bandage, always wrap from the most distant part of your limb toward your heart, which encourages the swelling to move up and away from the limb.
- **Elevation:** The last letter of RICE, e, is for "elevation" and really pertains to when an injury has swelling. An example would be if you turned your ankle running. In this case, if you elevate your foot above your heart while lying on the couch, it will help reduce any swelling.

REAL MOMS RUN

Some days running sucks and you think, *why am I doing this,* and so you stop and take the day off. Then the next time you run you feel that euphoria, and you feel all the stress just float off behind you, and you think *this is why I do this.*

—Julia, 29, two kids

The Dos and Don'ts of Injury Management

Do:

- Take a few days rest and see if the pain subsides.
- Cross-train only if the exercise doesn't aggravate the area.
- Seek the advice of a doctor that specializes in sports medicine or a physical therapist.
- Complete the recommended rehabilitation until cleared to begin running by the professional.

Don't:

- Run through pain.
- Alter your gait to avoid the pain.
- Tell yourself it will go away and ignore the symptoms.
- Take NSAIDs (nonsteroidal anti-inflammatories such as aspirin or ibuprofen) unless your sports medicine professional recommends it. They may temporarily relieve the pain but not address the problem.
- Self-diagnose your injury by searching the web. There is a wealth of information from reliable sources on running injuries, but Dr. Google isn't physically evaluating you. Get the correct diagnosis from a reputable sport professional first and follow her protocol.

You Shouldn't Run If . . .

- You have a fever or are dizzy or lightheaded.
- Your head is pounding, sinuses are swollen, or your nose is so stuffed that you are having difficulty breathing.
- Your child is so sick that your running will compromise her care.
- Your lungs are filled with congestion, so much so that your breath is gurgle-y.
- There is sleet, freezing rain, or the roads are icy and unsafe.
- An injury is bothered by running.
- You have the flu.
- Your doctor told you not to run.

RUNNING INJURIES

If you have just started running, are returning from a long layoff, or have changed the speed, distance, or terrain of your running route, it is common to be sore. Understanding the difference between sore and injured will determine if time off and attention is needed or if you can continue running. Soreness is normal for athletes and is a body's response to overload or fatigue. When you push yourself safely, your body responds by being sore—stiffness, achiness, and general muscle tenderness occurs. Typically soreness occurs bilaterally, meaning that both legs and body parts exercised are involved. Soreness is the body's way of repairing muscles and adapting to the new level of stress or exercise. Soreness can occur shortly after a run or up to twenty four hours later and last for several days. This is your body's repair mechanism, and soreness, while it may not always be comfortable, is perfectly normal.

An injury will have one or more of the following symptoms:

- Tenderness that is specific to one spot
- Swelling and extreme tenderness
- Pain in the tendon, joint, or bone
- Pain that alters your running gait

RUNNING INJURIES DECONSTRUCTED

Running injuries can span from simple to very complicated and complex. As a beginning runner, if you build slowly as you train for a 5K, hopefully you will never have to deal with anything major. However, things don't always go as we plan, so here are a few common injury descriptions and suggested treatments. This is simply advice from a fellow runner, but you should always seek your physician's medical attention any time you are in doubt about a niggle or an injury, and certainly for anything more serious, like a pulled muscle or a stress fracture. Most running injuries occur because of muscle instabilities and imbalances. Using the Pick Six Strength Program, the proper warm-up and cool-down will help prevent these injuries from occurring.

Plantar Fasciitis

The plantar fascia is a thick band of connective tissue that begins at the base of your toes and runs the length of your foot to your heel bone. When the plantar fascia is stressed by overuse or a sudden increase in mileage, it gets angry and inflamed and becomes plantar fasciitis (PF). PF can also be the result of tight calf muscles and Achilles tendons, and can be caused by improper footwear. If you wake up in the morning and your first steps are painful, or if pain increases as you stand on your tiptoes, it is likely PF.

Treatment: Consult with a sports podiatrist, orthopedist, or physical therapist for the exact care and to determine the cause of the PF. Make sure you are not running in old shoes with a lack of proper cushioning. Try stretching your feet out by flexing and extending your ankles in the morning before you rise to get blood flow into the tendon and then repeat several times a day. Stand facing a wall and place one foot against it, then perform a slight lunge toward the wall to stretch out the back calf muscle. Rolling the bottom of your foot on a golf ball may be uncomfortable at first but helps relieve pain as well. Try rubbing your foot along the rung of a chair while you are seated at the dinner table. The more you can get blood flow to that plantar fascia, the more opportunity it has to heal.

Achilles Tendonitis

Hilly terrain or speed work can aggravate your Achilles tendon, causing stress and leading to small tears and inflammation. If not addressed appropriately, scar tissue will build up, making the Achilles and calf less flexible and more susceptible to tearing or rupture.

Treatment: Use the RICE method, stretch your calf muscle, and perform self-massage several times a day to promote healing. Try inserting a heel lift into daily shoes to take the stress off the calf muscle.

Shin Splints

Shin splints is the term for any pain that afflicts the front of the leg, or around your shin bone. This is almost always caused by running too much, too fast, and too often. The scientific term is tibial fasciitis, and it is marked by inflammation of the muscles of the shin and surrounding connective tissue.

Treatment: Make sure your shoes fit, or replace them if they are too old, as a lack of cushioning may be causing your shin splints. Decrease the mileage and intensity of your runs until the soreness has gone away and emphasize calf raises and stretches.

Runner's Knee

The most common injury among runners, runner's knee, occurs when the kneecap doesn't track smoothly over its cartilage groove. Doctors believe that the angle in which the hips descend to the knees can cause the kneecap to run off track. Women are often more likely to suffer from runner's knee, thanks to wider hips and child-bearing bodies. It is marked by pain, stiffness, or swelling around or under the kneecap. It may feel crunchy, like there is gravel under your kneecap, when flexing or extending your knee.

Treatment: Icing will help if there is a spot that is tender. Using a neoprene leg sleeve that has a hole for your kneecap can keep the kneecap stable so that it tracks properly. A sports podiatrist can determine if your feet are over-pronating (rolling inward) and causing the mechanics of your gait to aggravate your knee.

IT Band Syndrome

Your iliotibial band runs from your hip along the outside of your thigh all the way down to your knee. This long strip of connective tissue is not flexible, so it cannot be stretched or strengthened. Iliotibial band syndrome (ITBS) usually begins with pain on the outside of the knee but can run the whole length of the outside of the thigh. Sometimes inflammation of a bursa at the hip will cause a snapping or popping that is painful while running.

Treatment: The muscles surrounding the IT band—the hamstrings, glutes, and quadriceps—can be strengthened and stretching these muscles will help alleviate ITBS. Try using a rolling pin to roll along your IT band or invest in a foam roller to help relieve the inflammation.

Hamstring Tendonitis and Piriformis Syndrome

Both of these injuries are literally a pain in the butt. Hamstring tendonitis involves the muscles that make up the backside of the leg from the knee to the pelvis. Piriformis syndrome affects the lower hip region. Both present in a similar manner, with pain on sitting, numbness, tingling down the leg, and pain while climbing stairs or running uphill. These two injuries also can feel like lower back pain, so getting in and out of your car and sitting for long periods might become painful.

Treatment: Avoid strain to the back and sitting for long periods. If you sit at work, make an effort to change positions, get up and walk every hour, and stretch during the day.

MUSCLE TEARS AND PULLS

Muscle tears and pulls are injuries that require time off and medical attention. If the injury happens in a traumatic way such as an ankle roll, slip, or as a pain that comes on quickly instead of slowly, it's time to stop and pay attention. Continuing to run with a muscle tear or pull will not resolve the problem. This is the time to consult a sports medicine professional who can devise a plan to get you back on the road in a safe, timely manner. Sudden injuries require careful attention.

STRESS FRACTURES AND THE FEMALE TRIAD

Most running injuries involve a muscle, tendon, or a ligament, but once in a while, the bone can also be involved, resulting in a stress fracture. A stress fracture happens as a result of increasing intensity and mileage too soon, before the bones have had time to adapt. Remember that weight-bearing exercise helps to keep bones strong by increasing bone density. If you increase mileage and intensity too quickly, the bone fails to keep up and microfractures occur. A stress fracture is typically marked by sharp, specific pain, not an all-over pain. Once diagnosed by a sports medicine professional, a stress fracture will need to be rested for three to six weeks, depending on the location of the injury.

A condition called the female athlete triad can affect women in all stages of life. Marci Goolsby, an assistant attending physician in the Women's Sports Medicine Center at the Hospital for Special Surgery in New York City, explains: "The female athlete triad is made up of three components: energy availability, menstrual status, and bone health. Energy availability refers to the amount of nutrition matching up with the energy that is expended. This doesn't mean that a woman has to have disordered eating to have low energy availability; she simply can be a busy mom that is paying more attention to what her children eat than what she takes in. The energy deficit throws off her hormones and makes a woman at risk of losing her period, called amenorrhea. This imbalance between nutrition and exercise affects your hormone access from your brain to your ovaries and in turn affects your bones, causing stress fractures and in the long term, osteoporosis. Many times the female athlete triad is not recognized because a mom is breastfeeding or is taking the birth control pill and so a normal period is not happening."

Dr. Goolsby's three key ingredients to injury prevention are strength training, appropriate nutrition, and calcium intake.

TEN RUNNING ANNOYANCES

Before any injury (or even a niggle) occurs, you are more apt to encounter a running annoyance. Most of these are minor, and easy to treat. You should be prepared to handle each one, as they will definitely come up at some point during your running career.

Black Toenails

Consider it a mark of a runner or use it to get a discounted pedicure. In most cases, a black toenail is totally preventable simply by making sure your shoes are properly fitted, lacing your shoes so that your foot isn't slipping, and keeping your toenails trimmed.

Blisters

An improper shoe fit is almost always the culprit. When shoe shopping try on the shoe with the socks you wear running. But sometimes, no matter the fit and sock, a runner is plagued with blisters. In this case, a smear of lubricant can ease the friction. If a blister appears, leave the skin intact, as it serves as a protective barrier until your new skin is ready.

Breast Discomfort

As long as you wear a supportive running bra designed for high-impact exercise, you should not be concerned that running is ruining your breasts. If you are bothered by the movement of your breasts while running, try doubling up on your sports bra or adding a compression-type fitted shirt to reduce bounce. If you are experiencing redness, indentation marks caused by the straps, or chafing around the rib cage, see the following.

Chafing

If you have experienced chafing, you know that the tiniest amount of friction can overtake your every thought until the run is over or the contact point is changed. Chafing is caused by the rubbing of body parts, such as between the thighs or arm to torso, or between a body part and clothing, such as bra to body or shorts to thighs. The sodium in your sweat can irritate an already raw, sensitive area. Petroleum jelly works as an excellent lubricant between body parts or between clothes and skin, or you can try BodyGlide, a sports lubricant that offers a greaseless, stainless alternative.

Callouses

If the manicurist looks up at you with horror as she begins your pedicure, it is because you are a runner. If it isn't the black toenail, then it is the callouses that the miles are putting on your feet. Another badge of honor, the callous happens because of your new sport and the repetitive movement in your running shoe. Refrain from cutting into callouses as you risk creating a blister or causing an infection. Callouses can be smoothed with a pumice stone. To keep your feet lovable, I recommend using pumice in the shower and then slathering your feet with a deep moisturizer, slipping on a pair of old socks, and wearing them to bed to lock in the moisture. Your partner may not think it is attractive, though he will appreciate the outcome the next night when silky smooth feet snuggle up to him.

Dehydration

If you are parched, drink water. Dehydration can cause muscle fatigue and loss of coordination, decrease performance, and lead to a heat-related illness. Maintaining good fluid intake in your daily routine by remembering to drink when you are thirsty should be enough to keep you hydrated. Most of the water that is lost while training for a 5K can be replaced after your workout.

Heat Illness

Heat-related situations can be very serious, but they are preventable if you use common sense when exercising and listen to your body. Heat illness can be as small and annoying as a cramp, and hydration is generally the answer. A heat cramp could be the first indication that a body is in more trouble, however, leading to heat exhaustion and heat stroke. Heat exhaustion is identified by heavy sweating; weakness; cold, pale, and clammy skin; fast, weak pulse; nausea; vomiting; or fainting and can be easily managed by moving to a cooler location, sipping water, and cooling the body with wet sponges or clothes. Heat stroke is identified by high body temperature (above 103°F); hot, red, dry, or moist skin; rapid and strong pulse; and possible unconsciousness. This requires immediate medical attention. Be careful when running on very hot days, and listen to your body when it's telling you to stop.

Side Stitches

Side stitches usually occur under the rib cage, where the diaphragm is located. A side stitch happens when you over-run your fitness level and your breathing can't keep up with the level of exertion you are demanding. To relieve a side stitch, slow to a more tolerable pace or stop running and walk until the pain subsides.

The Trots

This is a universally accepted running term for that immediate moment when your bowels decide you need to go, and now. Usually there isn't so much as a few minutes warning before the urge takes over your every thought and footstep. Panic makes the urge worse as you search your worldly options to relieve yourself. RIP (running-induced poop) occurs because of the bouncy nature of the sport combined with the lack of blood flow going to the intestine. If you run early in the morning, try waking up at least a half-hour before to hydrate and "move things out" before heading out the door. As a new runner, it may take time to understand your body and when it needs to go. Running does make you more regular, though it may take several weeks of a routine to figure it out. Don't be embarrassed if this happens to you on a run; every runner has had RIP at least once, so be proud you joined the ranks.

Tinkle Trouble

If you have given birth, have gone through menopause, or happen to be one of nearly 45 percent of women that suffer from urinary incontinence, running might be as exciting a venture as jumping on your children's trampoline. Even the mention of the word *tinkle* might evoke a dribble.

In running, the most common tinkle troubles involve stress incontinence, when the action of running causes urine to leak. Pregnancy, childbirth, and menopause can weaken the pelvic floor muscles, causing the urethra to be unable to shut off completely, and that is when tinkle "escapes." This causes leaking during moments of stress, like running, sneezing, or coughing. While it might be comforting to know that nearly half your friends may be suffering too, it doesn't fix the situation. If you suffer from bladder problems that are keeping you from living a regular life, it is time to see a doctor. There are many options to correct stress incontinence, and the easiest is incorporating Kegel exercises into your daily routine.

Kegel Exercise

As you are going to the bathroom identify the muscles you can contract to stop the flow of urine. These are your pelvic floor muscles, and this is the exercise you would like to replicate. Try contracting and relaxing those muscles for 5 seconds on and 5 off for a set of 10. Done daily, Kegel exercises will help strengthen the very muscles that are getting you into tinkle trouble. If you are still suffering from incontinence, discuss with your doctor the many other options she might have to help.

Running is a lifelong sport, provided you listen to your body and react to niggles if they arise. A few days off prevents a long layoff later if you pay attention to your body. Eating right, strength training, and monitoring your calcium intake are the building blocks to a sound body that can remain injury-free, and ready to race.

REAL MOMS RUN

I run because I can. I think the reason I run is different every single time I put my sneakers on. One day it might be to earn a nice glass of wine with dinner; another day it might be to shake the stress of work. The next day it might just be to test my limits about how far or fast I can run. That's the best thing about running—there are a million reasons why I do it and very few (okay, no) reasons why I shouldn't do it.

—Rebecca, 32, two kids

PART 3

See Mom Race

"The time has come. The time is now.
Just go. Go. GO! I don't care how."

—Dr. Seuss (from *Marvin K. Mooney Will You Please Go Now!)*

CHAPTER 8

Pre-Race Prep

Following the training program in Part 2 is the first step toward race preparedness, and when you do, I am certain that your body will be ready to compete in a 5K. Whether you run, run/walk, or walk briskly, you are doing the work necessary and your body will be ready to go. Just like pregnancy, you shouldn't go to a 5K race without understanding what to expect. And just like pregnancy, the best-laid plans do not always accommodate when something goes awry, yet the baby comes anyway. It is in times like this that we are truly tested, but with a little mental preparation you can adjust to any unforeseen situations and still be successful.

This race preparation is about you. Selfish as it is, *you* are competing in this 5K for you and you only. The expectations that you have should be your own—you need to own your race expectations so that you believe it can be done. Setting a running goal, what to wear, how to eat, getting enough sleep, and remaining positive are all part of preparing properly. When you register for a 5K, you should do it with the notion that you are challenging yourself in a healthy manner. You don't have to win, place in your age group, or come in the top of anything; you just have to cross the finish line knowing that you competed to better your body and mind.

SET A RACE-DAY GOAL

Oftentimes I hear women getting ready for a 5K say their goal is just to finish. Really? Don't you expect more of yourself than *just* to finish? This statement discounts your effort to move yourself forward, the weeks of training you have completed, and your sense of accomplishment. You *deserve* to finish, but you also deserve more. I am going to tell you now that *my* goal is for you to finish. *Your* goal will be to settle on a realistic time and then to cross the finish line as close to that time as possible with hands pumped and a smile across your face.

So how do you determine your goal time? During the weeks of training you became familiar with your conversation pace and how fast that is per mile. If you don't know how to do this, try doing your workout at a high-school track or map a route where you know the mileage. Divide the minutes of your workout by your mileage, and you will get your minute per mile pace. For example, if you are doing the Crawling Program and it takes you 45 minutes to do the run/walk portion (without warm-up and cool-down) and you covered 3.1 miles, your pace per mile would be 45 minutes divided by 3.1 miles, or a 15-minute pace. This is your training pace. If this is your first 5K, your goal can be your training pace and you will finish with confidence. Should you want the race to challenge your training pace, try taking 30 seconds off per mile of your conversation pace or about 1½ minutes off the 5K time. This should be enough to challenge yourself and finish strong. If you have raced in a 5K before, review your previous finish and compare your current fitness to the level you last ran to determine your best goal time. If the previous 5K was more than five years ago, you should consider this a new race distance and work off your training pace to determine a time.

PACE CALCULATOR

Mile Time	5K Time
6:00	00:18:38
7:00	00:21:44
8:00	00:24:50
9:00	00:27:56
10:00	00:31:02
11:00	00:34:08
12:00	00:37:14
13:00	00:40:20
14:00	00:43:26
15:00	00:46:36
16:00	00:49:42
17:00	00:52:49
18:00	00:55:55
19:00	00:59:01
20:00	01:02:08

Do not set a goal time that is too aggressive. If you are running a 10-minute mile at conversation pace, it is unrealistic to think you will finish the race at an 8-minute mile pace. During the weeks leading up to the race, you will learn your pace and capability. It is great to be optimistic in shaving off a minute per mile from your pace, but more than that could be disastrous and set you up for failure. Be smart and confident with your first time racing and you will be successful.

You can set a second goal if you feel that the course or weather may be disruptive to your primary goal time. If, for example, you have decided on a 30-minute 5K and then preview the course and notice it is hillier than expected, you might need a revised goal. Adding in a few extra minutes will allow you to tackle the hills without overdoing it for the rest of the race. Being able to adjust to race-day conditions will allow the flexibility you need to reach your goal.

Once you have the goal time, write it down and review it weekly to make sure you are comfortable and to keep you on task. Be proud, and tell your friends and family. Your declaration shows your commitment. You're not doing this *just* to finish. You have purpose, and you have worked hard.

REAL MOMS RUN

To be honest, every time I am at a race, I am inspired. I love seeing all walks of life come together to run. There are very few sports that can show that much diversity at one time!

—Amanda, 33, two kids

CHOOSE YOUR RACE-DAY OUTFIT

When you're deciding what to wear on race day, remember this play on an old English wedding rhyme: Something Old, Nothing New, Nothing Borrowed, Something Blue (but only if it's your color).

As you prepare for race day, it's not the time to experiment and try new clothes, new food, or different sleep patterns. Trust in what you have rehearsed prior to race day and have confidence in your decisions.

Some thought needs to go into your race-day attire, long before the morning of the race. If you have the budget, it is fun to buy a race-day outfit but it isn't necessary; the clothes you train in are more than acceptable. Make sure you wear your race-day outfit a few times before race day to make sure you are comfortable and there is nothing chafing or irritating. The littlest bother during a training run magnifies tremendously on race day. If you do decide to buy a new outfit for your race, take into consideration the following:

- **Comfort:** If it doesn't feel right in training, it won't feel right on race day. If it doesn't feel right in the dressing room, forget about it.
- **Weather:** Always check the forecast and be prepared for adverse conditions. If you are racing somewhere cool, it is best to dress in layers and peel them off as you warm up. Never wear something that is too hot and can't be adjusted. Plan your clothing as if it is twenty degrees warmer than the race-day temperature once you get moving. Keep in mind that nerves and early morning temperatures can make you chilly and a jacket may be necessary up until the race start.
- **Color:** Try wearing something that stands out such as a neon color or stripes so your friends and family can easily spot you in the crowd. Bright colors are festive and fun for 5Ks. The brightness will make others smile, which will in turn make you smile.
- **Ease of removal:** Make sure whatever you choose is easy to remove should you have to use the wonderful race-day port a-johns. Really, practice this. If you are inclined to wear a one-piece suit or something that requires additional time to get in and out of, this could be harmful on race day. Race-day nerves sometimes are expressed in race-day urgent needs to use a bathroom, and having to struggle with clothing in a tiny space is difficult.
- **Cotton is Rotten:** Regardless of the color or style, cotton is a difficult fabric to wear on race day. In a 5K, a cotton T-shirt shouldn't be a deterrent since the race is not long, but steer clear of cotton socks for any distance, especially if the race takes place in a hot, humid climate.

COLLECT YOUR RACE-DAY T-SHIRT

Most races give a commemorative race-day T-shirt with registration. This shirt is your badge of honor, and you've earned the right to wear it proudly. But should you wear it on race day? The answer is: sometimes and never. You should sometimes wear your shirt if there is a race-day tradition to wear it or if it is a themed race. My Run Like a Mother 5K, for example, is on Mother's Day, and traditionally people wear their shirts. It's fun to see a sea of one color celebrating the event. If you do decide to wear the race-day T-shirt to the race, try to pick it up days before the race so you can wash it and ensure that it fits properly.

Many seasoned runners believe that you should never wear a race-day T-shirt until after you have crossed the finish line. But even if you're not superstitious like that, remember: race day is not a time to find out something is bothersome by wearing a shirt that's uncomfortable.

If you want extra encouragement from the spectators, try writing your name on a piece of duct tape and put it across your chest. Make it big and bold. Shamelessly plugging your effort is good motivation!

EAT RIGHT FOR RACE DAY

You may have heard that you need to "carbo-load" before a race by filling your body with carbohydrate-rich foods several days before to provide muscles with enough fuel to finish strong. This practice is for endurance races that take over 90 minutes to complete. In a 5K race, you will be over and done before your body has the chance to run out of fuel, so it is not necessary to carbo-load or increase calories prior to race day. All the rules about eating while training that we went over in Chapter 6 apply to race week and race day too. Don't try anything new or experimental, and don't borrow a diet or food because it works miracles for a friend unless you have had time to test it.

Pre-Race and Race-Day Eating Tips

- The day before the race stay away from high-fiber and high-fat foods that can cause intestinal distress.
- Make lunch the largest meal the day before the race.
- Eat a light dinner that includes a lean protein and pasta or rice. My favorite pre-race dinner is salmon and rice.
- Hydrate well the day before the race. If it is going to be hot and humid on race day, try drinking a sports replacement drink (sixteen ounces or so), mixed

with water between meals to increase your sodium intake, which will help on race day.

- If you are traveling to a race, refrain from trying the local cuisine if your body is not accustomed to it. If you aren't familiar with the regional food, pack ready-to-eat foods that you are used to eating.
- Eat a light meal that is easily digested at least two hours before the race day. A favorite pre-race meal of many athletes is a small banana and half a bagel with peanut butter.

If you drink coffee in the morning, by all means, drink it. Allow yourself enough time to use the bathroom though, as hot liquids have a tendency to get things moving. If you are not a coffee drinker, race day is not a time to start.

If you don't typically run in the morning, have a few "rehearsals" with your food and body before race day. Try replicating the race day by waking and eating at least two hours before running to see how your body reacts.

GET YOUR ZZZS IN

Have you ever heard the saying "Sleep is not necessary for awesomeness"? It's a nice thing to remember before every race. Pre-race jitters steal sleep worse than a newborn baby. This is normal. Anxiousness can cause sleep disruption and crazy race dreams. You may find yourself dreaming of getting lost on the race course, forgetting your shoes, or even oversleeping and missing the race. These dreams (or nightmares) and disrupted sleep can cause worry and feelings of doubt. This is anxiety and is a normal reaction to stress. It is common to have a fitful night of sleep on race-day eve. If you accept the pre-race jitters as normal, it will make your race more enjoyable.

A 2013 Dutch study confirmed that athletes that experienced a lack of sleep before a performance actually covered the same distance in the same time as athletes that had normal sleep, though when interviewed the sleep-deprived athletes didn't feel that they performed as well. Their body performed the same; it was their minds that didn't believe it. Just try to get a normal night of sleep the few nights before the race. Whatever normal is for you is sufficient.

DEAL WITH DEBBIE DOWNER, NANCY NEGATIVE, AND ELLEN EXCUSE

Let's hope that the only mean girls you'll have to deal with on race day are Debbie Downer, Nancy Negative, and Ellen Excuse—those imaginary people who symbolize your worst thoughts and that can turn a race experience into a disaster. Negativity and self-doubt are normal in untested experiences such as your first 5K or even for a seasoned athlete who wants to perform her best. So much of self-doubt stems from incorrectly anticipating the future and worrying about it. What if I can't finish the race? What if I get a leg cramp? What if the sky falls down? We don't know what we don't know and spending time worrying about it causes tension and stress. Try to live in the present and embrace what you can control, which is most importantly a positive attitude. Instead of negative thoughts, try visualizing a relaxed, smiling self, enjoying the race and crossing the finish line with hands in the air and a success to celebrate. Debbie Downer, Nancy Negative, and Ellen Excuse can ruin your race, so you have to find a strategy that works for you to leave them behind.

How to Get Rid of Negative Thoughts

Dr. Alan Goldberg, director of the sports consulting firm Competitive Advantage, has a few tips for athletes about handling negative thoughts:

1. Avoid fighting with your negatives and try to turn them into positives.
2. Remind yourself that last-minute negative thoughts and doubts are normal.
3. Reassure yourself that you can still run your very best with them.

4. Understand that your response to the negatives is what's important here.

5. Immediately refocus your concentration on your pre-race ritual.

DON'T LEAVE RACE-DAY LOGISTICS TO RACE DAY

Most race day stress can be eliminated with thoughtful planning ahead of time. Here are a couple of things you can do in advance to make sure everything goes smoothly on the day of the race.

Pick Up Race-Day Gear Early

Most races allow you to pick up your race number bib and other goodies (known in the running world as "swag") a day or two before the race. If pre-race package pickup is offered, try to take advantage, as waiting until race morning can add unnecessary stress to your day. Larger races may have "race expos" with vendors selling everything from nutritional products to running shoes. It can be an electric atmosphere: athletes congregating to talk about the race, caught up in the running excitement, and surrounded by new and sleek products that promote faster running (or so they want you to believe). But these vendors are appealing to your inner doubt. Take a look around, and maybe you'll see something you like. But just remember: do not use anything untested (by you) on race day.

Know the Course

While some athletes prefer not to know what is around each bend, I recommend at least driving the course to familiarize yourself with the terrain, especially if it's your first race. If the race is local and you are able to run the course during your training, in bits and pieces or in its entirety, by all means do it. Do not run the course the few days before just to see if you can do it. Trust your training. Sometimes you won't be able to preview the course due to travel restrictions or for safety reasons. In this case, most races provide a course overview, many with elevation profiles and detailed descriptions on their website or race literature.

Lay Out Your Clothes

Just as your kids prepare for their first day of school by choosing an outfit (I used to sleep in mine), it is important to lay out your race-day clothes the day before the race. I recommend doing this the morning before race day to allow ample time to discover that something is missing. Start with your feet and work your way up. Make a checklist for yourself so you don't forget anything:

- ○ Shoes: Check to make sure there is a right and left, and that the laces are in good shape.
- ○ Socks: I always stick one in each shoe so I know they are accounted for and ready to go.
- ○ Shorts, skort, or other bottoms: If the weather is iffy, be prepared for alternative clothing. Bottoms are hard to take off in a race, so plan accordingly. It may be best to stay warm in pants right up until race time, then remove them minutes before the race and shiver a little before the start.
- ○ Running bra: If you are prone to chafing, use Vaseline or BodyGlide generously where straps have the potential to rub.
- ○ Shirt: If you have already picked up your bib, make sure it is securely fastened to your shirt.
- ○ Jacket: If it gets too warm, it can always be tied around your waist. It is always great to have a jacket handy after the race as you cool down.
- ○ Hat and sunglasses
- ○ Chap Stick, sunscreen, and other items
- ○ Post-race clothing

Set Alarm(s)

If you're not an early person, make sure you have an alarm set and maybe even a backup to wake you on race morning. Don't rely on a spouse or partner to wake you up because if he forgets, you might not forgive.

Eat Two Hours in Advance

Allow enough time to eat at least two hours before a race. If you tend to have a nervous gut before the race, you should likely allow a little bit more time to digest.

Wear Your Race Bib

A race bib is the numbered piece of paper given to you by the event that tells the race directors who you are, and it is how they capture your time. It also signifies that you are a paid entrant. No number? No racing. This is the most important piece of gear (besides your clothing) that you must wear on race day. Bibs are intended to be worn in the front, either pinned to your torso or worn on a race belt designed to hold a bib securely. If you plan to safety pin the bib to your shirt, make sure to do it so that it can be seen but also does not get in the way of your running. Secure it while the shirt is on your body. Most women will pin it directly under their bra line. Many races today are "chip-timed," and the bibs have a computer chip attached to the back that will record your effort and automatically determine your time as you cross the finish line. Because this computer chip may be on the back of the bib, it is important that you do not fold or crumple it. The bib is yours to keep as you cross the finish and is a fun memento from the race.

Plan Travel and Parking

Always arrive to the race at least a half-hour before it begins if you have already picked up your race-day goodie bag. If you are unable to pick up until race morning, then you should arrive at least an hour before the start to allow time to pick up the bag. Most races will have detailed instructions about best travel routes, especially if road closures keep athletes from getting to the start. If the race is a large race in a big city, consider taking mass transit to eliminate last-minute parking problems.

Find the Bathrooms

When you arrive to the start, find (and use) the bathrooms. Lines form quickly and waiting until the last minute might keep you from starting the race when the gun goes off. My race-day strategy is stand in line, tinkle, stand in line, and go again.

Line Up Appropriately

It is imperative that you place yourself in a spot at the start that is reflective of the pace you plan to run. Do not place yourself in the front of the 5K race start unless you are planning to run a 6-minute mile. Your race will be most enjoyable if you start with like-paced athletes. Many races will have pace markers to line up near to ensure you are starting in the correct place.

Soak It Up

Once you are cued in line and waiting for the start, look around and soak up the pre-race vibe. You earned the right to race through weeks of training, and now the race is the reward!

And, finally: Encourage your family to be there to cheer you on and welcome you as you cross the finish line! It is wonderful for your children to see you race and celebrate your accomplishment. Let someone else be responsible for their race-day logistics because this is your day.

REAL MOMS RUN

Running gives me a chance to just be me. I get to push pause on laundry, carpooling, homework, and all the other "Mom" stuff and go out and pound some pavement, or treadmill. I run because it helps keep those dark depression clouds away. Other than when my kids are hugging me there is not a better "sunnier" time for me than when I finish a run. On races my heart bursts with pride in myself as I high-five kids, get cheered on by strangers, and cross the finish line.

—Tracy, 35, three kids

CHAPTER 9

Finding Your Race-Day Groove

The ability to race well happens by being prepared both physically and mentally. You've spent six weeks preparing your body for the race, and now the big day is here. It is time to show you can do it, Run Like a Mother, and have some fun. In this chapter, you will learn how to start with the right attitude, and maintain it through the finish line. We'll put the final touches on race-day execution so that there are no unexpected surprises and arm you with the Dos and Don'ts (and a few Maybes) of racing.

FIND YOUR INNER QUEEN

In my hometown Run Like a Mother race, most of the looped course is kind, with gentle elevations that are attractive to first-time 5Kers, but then at about 2.5 miles, a time in the race that the finish line feels oh, so close, you come to a Mother of a Hill. Your legs are tired and your body is sweaty, but everyone keeps running with bountiful smiles, because when you get to that hill, you also get to Queen Noreen. She comes every year and cheers the runners up and over the hill on their way to the fast downhill run then right to the finish line. "You can do this," she beckons with balloons in hand at the crest of the big hill. Her voice and smile are contagious, and women look for her every year to nudge them to the finish line.

Even though there may not be an actual Noreen at your race, the cool thing is that we all possess a bit of her inside of us, and it is up to us to draw on that positive attitude for race day. Whether it is your first race or your six hundredth, everyone needs a little oomph, push, and attitude to get to the finish line. Even the most finely tuned athletes sometimes forget to believe in themselves and end up falling apart on race day. Because no matter how much we prepare physically, to truly feel ready you have to maintain a positive attitude and believe that you can do it. If you're having trouble, try to picture your version of Noreen standing at the top of the hill cheering you on, and yelling: "You can do this."

REAL MOMS RUN

I am now wearing tutus for my races. Why? Well because I run to have fun and a tutu makes everything that much more fun.

—Tracy, 35, three kids

STAY IN THE *NOW*

You can lose confidence when you start to worry about the future. What if I can't go up that hill? What if my leg develops a cramp? What if I don't finish the race? The what-ifs crush our optimism, and yet, they don't even exist. You are worrying about hypothetical scenarios that you can't control anyway. It's easy to get absorbed by everything else that's going on like the weather or other competitors. But instead, as you are preparing to run the 5K, and especially while you are out there on the course, keep your mind focused on what you are doing at the current moment. In other words: Stay in the Now.

When you are in the Now, you won't worry about what you can't do or what you can't control, because you're focused on what you can. Take in all that is positive and right in your race, and release anything that is negative. A sunny disposition makes for a solid effort. Even if you're a 5K pro, if you don't bring your belief in yourself and the ability to be in the present, you can fall apart on race day. So as you wake up and lace up on the morning of the race, think about what you can do, and think about your Now, you will always find your groove.

MAKE A PLAN

After reviewing the race course, whether by car or on foot, it is smart to visualize a race strategy. I know you are thinking: *Don't I just have to run?* That may be true, but going in with a plan helps you control the outcome. It is helpful to write down your race-day plan so that you can understand what you are going to accomplish. Take the 5K and break it into time or mileage segments. Make the race into three 1-mile accomplishments. You can do anything three times! Or break it into 10-minute efforts. A race distance becomes more tolerable when you are not overwhelmed by the magnitude of the larger goal.

For example, if you have been following the Crawling Program and are planning to take walk breaks, it is smart to schedule them. Decide beforehand that you will run for 5 minutes and walk for 1 minute. If your watch allows it, set the timer so that it will beep to alert you for the next interval. Or, if the race has water stations, perhaps you can decide to walk through those and resume running after. Or, take a 2-minute walk break every mile. Maybe your plan will be to run the entire 5K but start with an 11-minute pace for the first mile, walk a minute, then progress to a 10-minute pace, again walking for a minute, then continue running and steadily building the pace as the finish line nears. Thinking about your strategy and writing out your race expectations help build your confidence. Remember, you can always make changes on race day with more walk breaks or whatever else you might need to do for a successful race.

START SLOW AND BUILD

The most successful races are accomplished by starting out slow and building into speed. Once the gun goes off, it is easy to get caught up in the commotion as your heart rate and pace soar in a "fight or flight" response of adrenaline. Expect this to happen, but try to be the tortoise, not the hare. Slow and steady will bring your heart rate up slowly and allow you to get stronger as you run. Use the first mile of the race to work into your pace and find your groove, maintain it during the second mile, and when you get to the third, you can really move.

DON'T COMPARE YOURSELF WITH OTHERS

There will be sinewy, trim runner bodies warming up all around you at the start of the race. Enjoy looking but don't worry about them. This is your race, your day, and you will do it in your body. If your friend is shamelessly promoting her agenda for the race, resist the temptation to think for a minute that you should be doing what she is doing. If you have made your plan, stick to it and don't be influenced or intimidated by others. Trust your training.

Have a Mantra

When you are training or racing and your mind begins to wander from Now, a good mantra can bring you back into focus. Play around with words and phrases that motivate you and then draw on them when you start to lose focus. Choose a phrase that you believe in and try repeating it to calm your thoughts. Here are a few examples:

1. Strong. Smooth. Steady.
2. I came here to run, and I will do this.
3. 3.1 has nothing on me.

4. I am a runner. I am running. I will finish.
5. Cool head, warm heart, hot legs.
6. Just keep running, just keep running, just keep running.
7. I'm lean. I'm fit. I'm strong.
8. Embrace, endure, enjoy.
9. Powerful, graceful, effortless.
10. Right foot, left foot, whole body runs.

EXPECT THE UNEXPECTED

There may be a time when, regardless of your positive effort, a race won't go as planned. Unforeseen circumstances happen and can be difficult to overcome. If you start to see your goal slipping, try to regroup. If this is your first 5K, you have so much to be proud of and the experience will give insight into the next race. Here are a couple of things to think about that might help:

- Focus on moving your knees forward: When you are finding it hard to hold your pace, think of putting one leg forward, then the next. Imagine your legs as pistons moving in rhythm. Count your steps to fifty then repeat. Counting will distract your thoughts and your steps will fall into place.
- Look ahead and find runners to pass: Make a plan to reach the woman in the red shirt, and then walk to the blue shirt, and so on. Your confidence will build as you pass others.
- Think of childbirth and know that this is easier: If you have given birth, a 5K is a walk in the park. Dig deep and breathe!

DOS, DON'TS, AND MAYBES ON RACE DAY

Do:
- Thank a volunteer: It is your day to shine, but without the many volunteers it wouldn't be happening.
- Smile: It says confidence and will relax you and the recipient.

- Be patient and tolerant of others: Races can bring out the worst in athletes. Long lines for registration or bathrooms can be frustrating. Don't waste your precious energy getting upset. Roll with it.
- Take walk breaks: Sometimes a little regrouping is enough to refresh your mind and body to complete the task in front of you.
- Drink water when you are thirsty: A 5K race will typically have one or two water stations. Make sure you are on the correct side of the road before you reach the water station. Don't dart or reach in front of another athlete. Make eye contact with the volunteer so that she knows you are going to take her cup. Do not come to a complete stop. Continue walking or running through the station. The best way to drink from a paper cup while moving is to pinch the top closed to form a small spout. Races like this typically have a "toss zone" where you can throw the cups onto the ground. If the cup still continues liquid, make sure you aren't dumping it or tossing the cup on another athlete.
- Give it all you got: Starting the race slowly and building into your pace is the smartest race strategy. Once you are in your groove, remember that *you* are in a race. A race is a competition and you are in it to win it, for you and no one else. Push yourself so that when you cross the finish line you feel like you accomplished the 5K effort to the best of your ability.
- Look up as you cross the finish line: This is your moment. Lift your head up, thrust your arms in the air, and take that memorable photo! You will always remember that feeling. If you are wearing a watch and timing your race, don't look down as you cross the finish line to stop your watch. Almost all races are timed, and they have your exact second recorded. Many races will even have it posted to the Internet within seconds of your finish. Take that moment to look up and smile, because you did it.

Maybe:
- Run with a friend: This is your choice, but I have always felt strongly that on race day, you should give your partners a hug at the start and then lose them in the crowd. Train with partners, but race for yourself. Never let someone's pace rule your race. You have trained for this day to see what you can do, and you should race knowing that at the finish it was all you.

- Wear headsets: If the race-day rules clearly state that headsets are not allowed, then do not wear them. Even when races allow headsets, be courteous and keep your volume at a level that you can hear what is happening around you. Also, your fellow runner may not share your taste in music, so kindly keep the music to yourself.

Don't:

- Bring a dog or stroller (unless the race says it's okay): You can train with a dog, and a stroller, but neither is appropriate on race day. While both may seem harmless to you, your fellow competitor might not find it too amusing to jockey for position with a wheeled or four-legged friend. Races that do allow strollers or animals generally will ask that you line up at the back of the start so you don't interfere with other runners.
- Sneak into a race without registering: Sneaking into a race without paying is stealing, and it's illegal. If you were shut out of registration for a race you really wanted to do, you just have to wait until next year or volunteer.
- Borrow a friend's bib: Your friend paid for the race and now has a wedding to attend instead. Why can't you just take her bib number? Imagine for a moment two scenarios:

  » You cross the finish line with a best ever performance, but the time is recorded in someone else's name. The local newspaper is there and snaps your photo to put on tomorrow's front page and your kids are thrilled. It's your photo and your friend's name in the caption. You are an imposter.

  » You are having the race of your life wearing your friend's bib, when suddenly a dog gets loose on the course and trips you. Now you are being whisked away by a medical person that is reporting your information to the med tent using the registered name of the athlete. Part of your race entry fee pays for the event organizer to insure the course and the registered runners, but that's not you.

- Line up in the wrong starting area: Stage yourself in the race according to your projected pace and finish time. Some races will have "corrals" or signs designating pace. This is a helpful way to ensure you seed yourself with runners of your same ability. Some will even assign your bib number according to your projected race time. If there isn't a designation, take notice of the athletes around you and seed yourself accordingly. If this is your first race and you don't know where to line up, start toward the back of the pack. This will prevent you from starting too fast and also give you confidence as you pass others.

- Pee behind a bush: Don't be that girl. Just don't be that girl.

POST-RACE TIPS

Congratulations! You have crossed the finish line, but your race does not end there. It's time to celebrate your run in a way that will maximize a nice recovery.

Walk

Don't come to a complete stop at the finish line, and refrain from sitting too quickly. Treat the race like a training run and do a cool-down, carefully bringing your body back to normal. If your family is excited to see you, encourage them to walk with you so that you don't come to a complete stop. After your walk, stick around the finish area and cheer other athletes in, share stories with other runners, and bask in the post-race celebration!

Refuel

You earned it. Most races will provide healthy recovery foods such as fruit, bagels, or energy bars. Check the race details before the race to see what is provided. If the pickings are slim, bring your own post-race nourishment; your body will appreciate the reward.

Stay Warm

Bring a jacket and sweatpants to throw on after the race. Even if the temperature is warm, your body cools down rapidly and sweaty clothing can chill you. Your muscles will appreciate the protection!

Wear Your Medal or T-Shirt

Be proud of your accomplishment. There is no shame in getting a little recognition. You earned the right to wear your medal and race-day T-shirt, so wear them the next day or all week if you like.

Walk the Next Day

The day after the race is evaluation day. You should take time to identify how you feel, where you are sore, if you ran the race you envisioned, and what you would have done differently. Take time the day after to go for a walk and reflect on the experience. Your body will be happy you are moving. This is called active recovery: bringing blood flow back to your muscles so the soreness can dissipate. Don't be too anxious to start running too quickly. Give your body a few days off with active recovery before ramping up your mileage.

REVIEW AND REPEAT

Once you have completed your first 5K race, give yourself a few days to assess your experience. Maybe you are already searching the Internet for the next 5K race, want to train for a 10K, or are recruiting your friends to train along with you. Maybe you never want to race again. Whatever your reaction is, take some time to really take it all in. Just like childbirth, sometimes the further away you get from the experience, the easier it is to imagine doing it again. Many people keep a journal to write down details about the race, how they felt while they were running, and also what they ate, how they slept, and to make notes about what they might do differently. It's also a good way to access thoughts you didn't realize you had about the experience.

REAL MOMS RUN

So much of my life is spent "running" errands, "running" children to activities, and "running" back and forth to work. Running is time I have found to spend all by myself, doing something for me. I feel that it has made me a better person. It has given me confidence in my own abilities, and I am happy to set a positive example for my family.

—Jennifer, 39, two kids

CHAPTER 10

The Finish Line

You've trained, you've made your goals, and you've run in your first, or maybe you're second, third, or thirtieth 5K race, but that's not the end of this story. For your training, and for your race, the focus has been on you, and rightfully so. Your responsibility to your fitness goals is only to yourself. But now you're officially in the club, and a part of the running community too. We don't have any hazing rituals (at least no official ones), but one thing I've always felt as a runner was this desire to pay it forward, encourage others to take their physical fitness seriously, and give back where I can. Here are a few ways to pay it forward. I hope they will inspire you to do the same.

RUN WITH YOUR KIDS

In 2010, First Lady Michelle Obama launched an initiative to combat childhood obesity. Let's Move! addresses the concern that children born after the year 2000 have a one in three chance of becoming overweight or obese. Mrs. Obama is dedicated to "ensuring that every family has access to healthy, affordable food. And, helping kids become more physically active."

The initiative offers an incredible idea: Train as a family for a charity walk or run. There it is, plain as day. Get your kids involved.

Many adults today are investing in their own health and leaving their children behind. If your child does not participate in afterschool organized sports, someone needs to make sure they move, and if you are the primary caregiver, that someone is you. Today, many children do not take the initiative to go outside and play because gaming devices and smartphones are so much easier. It is often hard to think of coming home after a long day to exercise our own bodies, and then to encourage your child to move. It can be a great opportunity for you to have an active conversation with your kids. Just as running with a spouse offers a unique opportunity to talk, running alongside your children opens up dialogue that needs to come out.

As you embark on your training, share with your children your plans and your goals. Share with them what you learn through each chapter, and make it your morning conversation. Integrate it into your life and it will become part of theirs too. Another great way to integrate running into your children's lives is to actually take them with you when they're still babies.

Running with a Baby Stroller

You can run with a traditional stroller up to a certain pace, but unfortunately they are typically built with a shorter wheel base and smaller wheels to make them easier to transport and navigate smaller spaces. At a faster pace, it will be harder to turn a traditional stroller, and the ride will be much bumpier than a running-specific stroller. Initially, a jogging stroller can be very expensive (they retail anywhere from $150 to $500 depending on the brand and the store), but if you are committed to running, it will last you a few years, and the overall investment is far less than a gym club membership.

Training can be a bit of a challenge at first as you learn to navigate the jog with your child in front of you, but there are a couple of things you should remember. Jogging strollers can usually carry a child from infancy (always check with the manufacturer to be sure) to about elementary school before she outgrows it (at about roughly

70 pounds and up to 44 inches in height). Double strollers, while more cumbersome to run with, can typically carry up to 100 pounds. Running with a jogging stroller takes a bit to get used to, but your running will quickly adjust. As your child grows and you push more weight you will become a stronger runner, particularly if you live in a hilly area. Make sure you are always going against traffic if you are running on the road, and it is very important to make eye contact with the driver of an oncoming car. And, as always, plan ahead for unforeseen circumstances. Bring an extra pacifier in case the first gets tossed, make sure you have extra diapers because you never know what can happen (the jiggling can get to the best of us), and make sure you have extra snacks (Cheerios are always an easy go-to), since all this running can work up an appetite for both you and your child.

Advantages of a Jogging Stroller

- **Wheel base:** Jogging strollers are typically built on a longer wheel base and have larger bike-type wheels, which allow for a smoother ride and better maneuverability. The three-wheel base makes the ride much smoother and allows you to lift the front wheel easily over bumps or uneven surfaces. This configuration also makes it easy to tip backward, so take care when you're on an incline or hanging things on the back if your hand is not there to support it. They can also be more cumbersome and harder to break down for storage, but the ride for the child and run behind are worth the inconvenience.
- **Safety:** Jogging strollers come with a leash or tether. This leash slips easily over your hand and keeps you connected to it just in case.
- **Brakes:** Jogging strollers have hand brakes (and also the standard wheel brake) that allow you to stop the stroller quickly. This is also helpful when running downhill to slow the stroller to a comfortable pace.
- **Comfort:** Your baby will be riding in a limo built for running. Jogging strollers today have a cockpit designed for your tiny bundle, with five-point harnesses, standard safety features, ample sun canopies, options for weather covers, and pockets galore. If your child isn't rocked to sleep by your pace, he certainly will have plenty of places to stash his books and gadgets to stay occupied.

When Is a Child Ready to Run with You?

As your children become more mobile and grow out of the stroller, it may become more difficult for you to take them along with you. They may want to run alongside you, but will likely have difficulty keeping up with your pace. Running as a young child is best if it is done in the form of play: informally in games like tag, steal-the-bacon, or duck, duck, goose, or in formally organized sports like soccer, lacrosse, or basketball. The Let's Move! initiative says school-aged kids should be getting 60 minutes of exercise a day. It sounds like a lot until you start to keep track of the time they may spend sitting at school, playing an electronic device, or watching TV. In a 2010 CDC review of fifty studies spanning twenty-three years, it showed that children who are physically fit perform better in a classroom than those that aren't. All the brain benefits of running from Chapter 1 apply to any size person, from child to adult.

And if your kids seem interested in competing the way you are, many races have kid's runs before or after the main event. From Diaper Dashes to Fun Runs to actual timed road races, these kid's runs are a safe, great way to involve the entire family. When a child begins to ask to run with you, by all means take the time to go. The run should be fun for both of you, and if you notice your child struggling to keep up, then slow down. Kids can run up to 6 miles in a soccer game, but there are always stops, starts, rests, and recoveries. Pure running is different, so adjust to the needs of your child, and choose appropriate intervals and pacing. If a child expresses the desire to run a 5K with you, talk to your pediatrician first. She will have a good idea if your child is ready physically to cover the distance.

REAL MOMS RUN

Running has absolutely affected my life in a very positive way! I have learned a lot about what I am capable of even at this age. Running has that unique ability to make a good day great, a bad day better, a horrible situation able to be borne.

—Kristin, 43, five kids

RUNNING AND SPOUSES

It can be the best of times and it can be the worst of times or sometimes both jumbled into one. I have seen couples running together, stride for stride, deep in conversation, almost as if they are in a bubble insulated from their surroundings. I have also seen couples running twenty feet apart, disengaged and annoyed, with resentful looks on their faces. I have seen marriages happen because of a mutual love of running, and I have seen marriages dissolve because of a one-sided love of running. Sometimes it is running bliss and occasionally it is a running mess.

If your spouse already runs, then lucky you. You already have a partner that understands getting up early, following a training schedule, the importance of a good night's sleep, and how to juggle life to wedge in a run. A running spouse will be excited to share his love, as runners live to convert non-runners. He may not want to run with you, or you may not be ready to run with him, but if and when you are fortunate enough to run together, it can be a magical date time—one that requires no makeup, money, or reservations.

I have always felt that difficult conversations with family members are easier when I am driving as they can share their thoughts and emotions without having to look me in the eye. It is the same with running. Otherwise touchy topics can be shared on the neutral ground that running provides. Running time together can be just the staple a marriage needs to discuss topics that can't be shared in a house full of little ears.

Though, as idyllic as it may seem, running with our spouses doesn't always work. Either our schedules don't permit the time away together, or our spouses simply don't run. Not every partner finds a new running habit exciting. However, the next best thing is a partner who tolerates and supports your running, and is cooperative when you need him to be. These are a few tips to help things go as smoothly as they can:

- **Involve him in your training:** Review your training schedule for the week with him. It is a team effort to balance a family, work, and recreation. Work together to find the time to fit in your runs in a way that he doesn't feel infringed upon.

- **Be honest with what running does for you:** If running makes you more productive, healthy, less stressed, and makes you a better mom, wife, and person, make sure you communicate this with your partner. It is likely that he will notice your physical changes, but it doesn't hurt to reiterate the positive emotional effects too.

- **Find a race that has great post-race atmosphere:** Look for races that offer a fun post-race party. Spouses are more inclined to support events with the lure of post-race beer or food. Chose races that are easy for your family to maneuver around; if your husband is coming with three kids and a stroller, a race that starts in one area and finishes in another (called a point-to-point race) won't be easy to navigate. Consider parking and ease of getting to the finish line when selecting a race.

- **Find a destination race:** Plan a vacation around a goal race or vice versa, and everyone is happy. You get to run and the family gets to play.

- **Support his interests:** If he has other interests, be supportive and accepting. You don't have to be passionate about the same activity, but being mutually supportive of each other prevents resentment about time away.

THE HALLOWED GROUND OF GIRLFRIEND RUNNING

While I love my husband and my daughters, there is nothing that can replace the running time that I spend with my girlfriends. I would do anything for my running friends, we share everything, and I am protective of this time together. The roads we have traveled and miles covered are sacred.

Earlier we discussed the importance of recruiting friends to train with because we are always more motivated when we have troops that support us. It may start with running dates with a few neighbors getting together to train for a 5K, but then morph into a weekly routine that transcends the goal. As you become more conditioned and comfortable with running at a conversation pace, the chatter will start to flow, even if there are awkward silences at first. My friends and I share a trust that rivals a patient-therapist relationship. Training plans come and go, but running with friends will carry you through every stage of your life.

Running Etiquette

When you run with training partners, you become very comfortable very fast, and this is never more apparent than when it comes to some of our less than ladylike bodily functions. You may bristle at the thought when you start, but you will be surprised what becomes acceptable once you become a more seasoned runner. Here's some of the proper etiquette for handling these delicate situations:

1. The Farmer's Blow: Running with a stuffed-up nose is not fun and chances are, you're not carrying a lot of tissues with you. So to get that mucous out of your nose on a run, it's important to master the Farmer's Blow. Make sure no one is behind you, and push one finger against the unaffected side to close the nostril. Turn your head to the affected side and either tuck your face down toward your armpit or over your shoulder. Blow with a quick force out of

the affected nostril (a tender blow will only be messy). Repeat with the other nostril if necessary.

2. **Tinkling in covert locations:** It is illegal in most municipalities to urinate in public, and I am not suggesting or encouraging such behavior. That being said, there are times when a quick dash into the woods has to happen. When nature calls, be on the lookout for property lines, poison oak or ivy, and animals. Look in all directions before squatting; you may be protected by one direction only to have headlights beam at you from another. If you are in an urban area, try to search out a public restroom first. If none exists, ask politely at a store and offer to come back and support their business just as soon as your run is over.

3. **Toot-toot:** No matter how hard you may try, there will be times that you can't prevent fluffing, poofing, breaking wind, or passing gas. Remember, running gets things moving intestinally, and so it is natural. It's up to you and your gang whether or not this is spoken of, but know that a good laugh and comment about the barking frogs will ease an awkward situation.

RUN ONE, VOLUNTEER ONE

A great way to stay energized and motivated to run is to volunteer at a race. It is an incredibly rewarding experience and it's a give-back for every time you've crossed the finish line. Whether they are for profit or for a cause, almost all races are organized and run by volunteers, because it takes a tremendous amount of effort to make these events happen. Most race volunteers share a love of running, and volunteering can be a super way to find training partners, learn about a race you might be interested in, and get discounted entries to future races. And, of course, most races will give you a race-day volunteer shirt, so if for no other reason, you will gain another shirt for your drawer. To get involved you can usually contact a race directly, or if you're having no luck there, reach out to local running clubs, since they usually have the skinny on these things. My motto is Run One,

Volunteer One, because it keeps me involved and reminds me why I love to race.

RUN LIKE A MOTHER

Do you remember when that first baby came into your life? How scary it was to bring home a tiny bundle that took over every waking thought, consumed your sleep, and monopolized the quiet moments? Now, months or years later, you can't imagine your life without the added child chaos. Running does the same thing. At first as your body struggles to acclimate, running feels uncomfortable and awkward. You are sore and out of sorts but also excited at the new regimen and potential of wellness. You shift your schedule to make room for it, open up time that perhaps never existed, and dive into running just as you did when your baby came home. Running is all-consuming at first. Your family may roll their eyes at your new-found love with the endless chatter about shoes and goal times, but soon enough they will see the transformation. They see the changes in your body and how it makes you a better mom, partner, and human being. Your running routine broadens your life. Even though it takes time that you thought you never had, it gives it back with renewed energy and efficiency. Running becomes who you are and what you do.

You are now armed with all the know-how to make running a part of your life, and it's up to you to figure out what to do with that. There's not much to separate you from making running a part of your life. The ability and the road are right there in front of you. Running will fill the crevices in an already full mother's life. It will strengthen your body and nourish your soul, and at the end of the day you will sleep better knowing that improving your life improves your family's life tenfold. Run Like a Mother. It's who you are. It's what you do.

REAL MOMS RUN

My son has taken notice of my running lately. The other day, he asked me, "Mom, can I run with you?" While us moms are always serving, picking up, and correcting our kids, I think sometimes that overshadows the bigger picture of what a mother can do—make a difference in our children's lives, each and every day. The fact is that they do see what you're doing, and you do have the power to inspire your children to be lifelong runners, to be lifelong achievers, to live healthy lives, and to believe that anything they put their mind to, they can do.

—Amy, 43, two kids

Index

ABOUT THE AUTHOR

Megan Searfoss is a wife and mother of three daughters who learned to run because she found it an inexpensive, time-saving, and mostly mind-saving exercise. She began running at age thirty when her oldest daughter was two, juggling motherhood, a career, a home, and everything in between. Now nearly twenty years and more than twenty marathons and numerous 5Ks, 10Ks, and triathlons later, she has found that a life with running has helped balance the chaos of work/life and brought self-fulfillment that she could have only imagined all those years ago.

A Health Coach; Personal Trainer; and Run, Cycling, and Triathlon Coach, Megan has participated in two Ironman World Championships, 2008 and 2010, in Hawaii.

While an elite athlete herself, Megan lives an ordinary life, with ordinary demands. She knows firsthand how challenging it can be to juggle the constant demands of work and motherhood, while still trying to find much-needed time for yourself. In an effort to introduce other women to the joy of running, she formed Run Like a Mother in 2008. What started as a small local race in Ridgefield, Connecticut, quickly grew to a national 5K race series designed to encourage women of all levels and abilities to experience the gift of running as a means to finding balance in their lives. By emphasizing simple training programs and practical lifestyle tips instead of technical overload, Megan has been successful at converting the skeptics into lifelong runners.

Running has been Megan's salvation through a time when all three of her daughters and her husband were diagnosed with Crohn's disease. She learned through her running that testing her body physically strengthened her mentally and allowed her to deal with life's twists and turns. For this reason coaching other women has been so rewarding: knowing that a strong heart makes a strong mind.

ABOUT RUN LIKE A MOTHER

Founded in Ridgefield, CT in 2008, Run Like a Mother was conceived to celebrate and empower all women: mothers, grandmothers, daughters, sisters, aunts, and friends—runners and non-runners alike. The race was a success, with more than 400 runners signing up in just five weeks. It has since grown to eight races throughout the country and is open to hundreds more who participate "virtually" across the world. Run Like a Mother also features an active online forum that offers daily support and advice for women on how to live a healthier, more fulfilling life.

The mission of Run Like a Mother is to fuel a woman's journey toward health and wellness; empower with education and training programs; inspire with communities, events, and races; and enable through programs and partnerships. Run Like a Mother Isn't Just a Race, It's Our Way of Life.

For more information, contact us at *info@runlikeamother.com.*